GOOD PRACTICE IN CHILD SAFETY

Angela Dare

Stanley Tho

First published in 2000 by:
Stanley Thornes (Publishers) Ltd
Ellenborough House
Wellington Street
CHELTENHAM
GL50 1YW
England

00 01 02 03 04 / 10 9 8 7 6 5 4 3 2 1

A catalogue record for this book is available from the British Library.

ISBN 0–7487–4502–5

Cover photo: Angela Hampton, Family Life Picture Library
Line illustrations by Jane Bottomley and Oxford Designers and Illustrators

Typeset by Columns Design Ltd, Reading
Printed and bound in Great Britain by T.J. International, Padstow, Cornwall

CONTENTS

ABOUT THE AUTHORS

The authors come from a background of health visiting, midwifery and teaching and worked together for many years at City and Islington College on a variety of child care courses. Angela Dare is currently an External Verifier for CACHE courses. The authors have published four books on child care topics.

ACKNOWLEDGEMENTS

The authors gratefully acknowledge the guidance and help they received from those who reviewed the first draft of the book. They also wish to thank Dominic Dare, Teresa O'Dea and Ursula O'Donovan for their help in researching various topics; also Christine Hobart, Victoria Tomking and Francesca O'Brien; and Helen and Jo Gallagher for the photographs of friends and family used within the text.

The Publishers gratefully acknowledge the following for permission to use copyright material:
The Stationery Office (pages 44 and 131). Crown copyright is reproduced with the permission of the Controller of Her Majesty's Stationery Office
NSPCC (pages 122 and 172)
CACHE (pages 80 and 135)
Child Growth Foundation (page 176)

INTRODUCTION

This book covers a variety of child safety topics. There are chapters providing information on accidents and accident prevention, safety in relation to child development, how to maintain a healthy and safe environment, responses to child abuse and an introduction to First Aid.

The book offers underpinning knowledge for child care students studying for CACHE and Edexcel (BTEC) Early Years courses, NVQ levels 2 and 3 and the Certificate in Child Care and Education. We feel it will also be helpful for workers within the child care field including Early Years and Key Stage 1 teachers, nursery workers, nannies and childminders. We hope parents may also find the book useful and interesting.

The principles of safety apply to wherever a child is cared for, whether the home, nursery or school. However, certain sections of the book address safety issues which are of particular relevance to specific settings and groups of children. The book aims to cover issues primarily concerned with children under eight, however some statistics cover data for children up to fifteen.

Legislation is subject to revision and amendment, so readers need to keep up to date with future changes.

Factual information is linked to good practice and Quick Checks. Activities are included to reinforce and extend learning.

1 CHILDHOOD ACCIDENTS

Child safety concerns not only the prevention of accidents but also the general protection of children from physical and emotional harm as well as the prevention of infection and diseases. Understanding the risks affecting children is not at all straightforward and many factors may combine to create potentially hazardous situations. Social circumstances, environmental hazards and the developmental stage of the child are all key factors in determining risk to any child.

Child care professionals have a responsibility to understand good practice in all areas of child safety and provide a secure environment in which children can grow and develop safely.

The importance of accidents

Accidents present varying degrees of danger to a child. About nine children die weekly as a direct result of preventable home and road accidents and, according to Home Office criminal statistics for England and Wales in 1996, approximately six children a year are murdered by a stranger (less than a one in a million chance). Yet, parents and society often focus more attention on 'stranger danger' than the very real hazards of home or road.

The Government can and does legislate for a safer environment. It is attempting to address the issue that children living in relative poverty are five times more vulnerable to accidents than children in more prosperous living conditions (*Our Healthier Nation: a contract for Health*, Department of Health, 1998). We increasingly use toys and equipment with recognised Safety Standard marks, and acknowledge the importance of adult supervision and attention when working with children. All of this, however, will not necessarily mean a child is safe unless we also understand her thought processes, reasoning and reactions. How we, as adults, interact and behave with a child is fundamental to her protection.

Accidents damage a child. The injury may be permanent or temporary, cause physical and emotional harm and sometimes even death. Indeed, apparently trivial accidents can cause pain, worry and anxiety to the child, her parents and carers. Most accidents can be prevented and no accident should be shrugged off as bad luck or a random event. Rather, every accident should prompt a reappraisal of child care practice, with a view to improving child safety. The leading national organisation concerned with child safety, The Child Accident Prevention Trust, feels that the term 'accident' should be replaced with 'unintentional injury' or 'injury accident' in a move to make people aware that 'unintentional injury' is, in fact, preventable.

Although deaths from accidents have declined in the last forty years, possibly as a result of advancing medical techniques, the number of accidents has not fallen significantly.

All research continues to tell us that a child under five is most at risk where she spends most time, usually the home, and a child over five most at risk on the roads. The adults most likely to cause her harm are family members or adults known to her.

CHILDREN'S VULNERABILITY

A child is vulnerable to accidents and injury simply because she is young, inquisitive and inexperienced. Her age and stage of development are linked to the numbers and types of accidents that happen. As a professional working with children, you undertake to provide an environment where they can grow, learn and thrive, protected from unnecessary harm.

A child constantly needs to practise her developing powers of reasoning, problem solving and judgement. She needs opportunity and support in developing muscle power, balance and control. When she is young, she will inevitably be clumsy, lack power, strength and deftness and will not understand about levels of risk. She has limited life experience on which to draw. She is unaware of the consequences of her actions in new situations. For example, a toddler does not understand that her cup which she turns upside down contains cold milk, while her mother's contains scalding hot tea, or that the grills over a fire remain hot long after the red glow has disappeared. She needs supervision and direction to learn as she grows.

A child's environment at home, nursery, school or outdoors is exciting and stimulating but full of potential hazards. She learns and develops rapidly. A baby is immobile one day but the next she can roll off a bed, then before long she can reach for dangerous objects, climb stairs, and open bottles. Parents and carers need to understand the changes and how quickly they occur, and plan for them.

The young child thinks accidents happen to others, and has little awareness of her own or any one else's role in keeping herself safe. As she grows, she needs to absorb and understand enormous amounts of complicated information quickly, for example, about walking outdoors and crossing roads. She will have to navigate through traffic, understand car speeds and distance, make allowances for driver unpredictability and be aware that a driver may not be able to see her

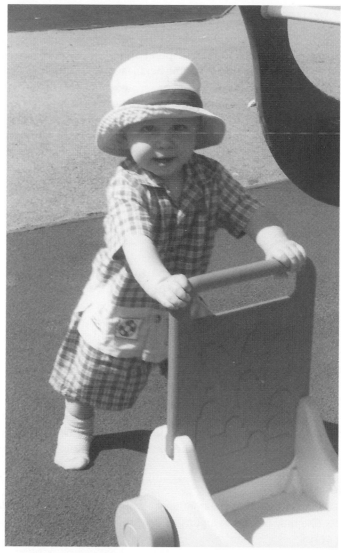

A child is vulnerable to accidents and injury simply because she is young, inquisitive and inexperienced

above a parked car. It is small wonder, then, that the road is dangerous and a child needs supervision until at least the end of primary school.

Consider the following.

- Babies under one have fewer accidents than children over five and those that occur are often the direct result of adults' careless actions.
- As a child grows, most accidents happen in places where there is less adult supervision.

KEY POINTS

- Carers need a sound knowledge of the developmental stages through which a child is proceeding and must respond appropriately.
- Anticipating and planning for the next learning or developmental stage is the key to safe practice.
- As adults, we must take responsibility to protect children when it is unreasonable for them to do this themselves.
- We must be constantly alert and respond promptly to environmental hazards.

REMEMBER

Anticipate changes, both environmental and developmental, and plan in advance.

Safety role models

Every adult and child is potentially a safety role model to another child. However, it is possible to unconsciously give unsafe messages. Young children learn by imitating and they have particular pleasure in copying the actions of adults and other children special to them. If, for example, you hurry across a road dodging cars rather than using a pedestrian crossing, or wander around drinking hot cups of coffee in children's play areas, children will consider this behaviour to be normal and will copy you. Your actions and explanations are the first lessons children learn, so it is important they see that you consider safety at all times and behave appropriately (see page 5). The closer your relationship with a child, the more influential will be your behaviour.

Older children in group situations often behave out of character and act in more dangerous ways than they would if on their own, for example, one child might 'egg on' another to climb higher and jump further in unsuitable situations, climb a frame with trailing clothes or run in dressing-up shoes on a wet surface.

REMEMBER

An older child often has great influence over her siblings and children in a younger group. She may behave in an unsafe way and unwittingly put these younger children at risk.

Overprotection

It may be impossible to entirely eliminate all danger and risk. If, in trying to create a completely safe world, you restrict a child's opportunity to discover and experiment, she will not learn. Overprotection may also prevent her from developing an understanding of risk – for example knowing whether an action is safe. Your anxieties will be transferred to her and she may become anxious and reluctant to make decisions and attempt new skills. This may affect her ability, confidence and enthusiasm to try new activities.

The outcome may be an increase in her vulnerability to danger: the child who is never given the opportunity to climb a low sturdy tree or frame fails to learn about balance, power and height estimation, to develop the muscles and

General

Be well rested. Get sufficient sleep
Do not abuse drugs or alcohol
Remember that the effects of alcohol can last well over 24 hours
Keep fit and eat a balanced diet to maintain high energy levels
If unwell, seek and follow medical advice. If you have an infection, absence from work may be necessary

Clothing

Wear unrestricted clothing that allows you to move freely, but without tripping or catching your heels
Wear well fitting, supportive and flexible low heeled shoes, with non-slip soles
Do not wear chunky rings or jewellery that can scratch and cut a baby or passing child

In addition

Keep colleagues and staff fully informed on changes to routines and children in your care
Update your own knowledge
Maintain a current First Aid Certificate

THE ROLE MODEL

Personal care

Have short clean nails
Keep hair out of your face and if necessary tie it back
Wear clean clothes daily and use fabrics that are easily laundered

Professional behaviour

Know the age and developmental stage of the children with whom you are working and plan your practice accordingly
Use equipment correctly at all times
Explain and show children how to use potentially hazardous tools e.g. scissors, knives
Clear up as you go and maintain a clean and tidy environment
Check daily the condition of small and large equipment, toys and play areas
Monitor daily the condition of the child's immediate environment – home, garden, school etc.
Be aware of a child with any special need and how the environment and equipment will need to be adapted.
Maintain:
- appropriate supervision levels
- a clutter free environment to limit tripping and falls
- a consistent approach to all safety matters

The child care worker as a role model

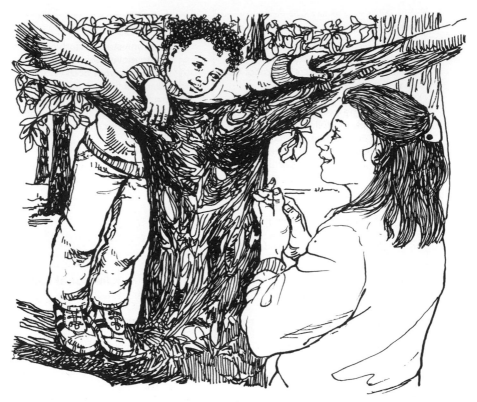

Offer suitable challenges, supervision and encouragement

strength necessary to pull and reach, and to experience the sense of exhilaration when she reaches her goal.

Instead she becomes nervous and clumsy, and when older and faced with similar challenges, she may avoid situations which demand such expertise or, conversely, take excessive and unrealistic risks. Children need to practise all their emerging skills within a controlled environment to boost their self-esteem and confidence.

REMEMBER

The occasional bump, bruise, minor cut or graze are inevitable when growing. However, nothing more serious should occur.

KEY POINTS

- Encourage children to develop and practise new skills.
- Help them to make safe decisions within a supportive and secure environment.

Family/Home

- Serious illness in family member
- Family carer tired, bored, affected by drugs or alcohol
- Family stresses, especially poverty, divorce
- Serious illness or disability
- Changes in routines e.g. moving house, holidays
- Poor knowledge of child development – unrealistic expectations of child
- Unsafe or unsuitable toys for developmental stage
- Highly disorganised household
- Low supervision levels/over-protective family
- Poorly maintained/overcrowded housing

School/Nursery

- Poorly maintained buildings including outdoor play areas and equipment
- Changing classes
- Friday afternoons
- Cluttered environments
- Low levels of supervision in high risk situations and areas e.g. playgrounds
- Mixed skill and age range groups

Child

- Tiredness
- Illness
- Hunger
- Certain disabilities especially visual and hearing impairments, dispraxia, learning difficulties
- Certain types of behaviour especially hyperactivity, shyness, excessive lack of confidence
- Inappropriate clothing, clothing too tight or too loose, shoe laces undone, shoes incorrect size

Carer

- New carer unused to child
- Poor practice
- Carer tired or affected by drugs or alcohol
- Carer under stress
- Limited knowledge of child care or developmental issues
- Disorganised
- Changes in routine
- Toys given unsafe or unsuitable for developmental stage of child

Society

- Low levels of maintenance of public buildings
- High traffic levels
- High traffic speeds
- Inadequate traffic calming measures
- Lack of suitable safe play areas
- High rise accommodation
- Lack of a 'child centred' attitude in society
- Inadequate support mechanisms for families under stress
- Low benefit levels to lone parents
- High costs of some safety equipment

General

- Seasonal factors
- Winter mornings and evenings when dark early
- Summer months for outdoor play
- Sunday evenings

Factors that contribute to increased risk

Factors which contribute to increased risk

There are many factors which can contribute to increased risk of accidents happening (see page 7). You must always plan a safe environment, use equipment in good condition with approved safety features, maintain adequate supervision and have a sound knowledge of a child and her development.

However, there will be times when accidents are statistically more likely to happen. Being aware of these times gives you the opportunity to make changes to minimise risk. Dangers are not always constant and hazards can change. For example, a child may be safe on the climbing frame today, but vulnerable tomorrow if her shoe laces are untied, if the frame is overcrowded or unstable or if several children with different skills are using the frame at the same time.

Activities

1 Look at the current and previous years' accident report books in your nursery or school. Clarify what is regarded as 'an accident'. It may vary from setting to setting depending on what is perceived as the severity of the incident.
   a) Look at the reports and consider the trends by observing:
      ■ the frequency of the accidents
      ■ the types of accidents
      ■ the time and day of the week an accident happened
      ■ where the accident occurred in the setting e.g. the playground, cloakroom etc.
      ■ the sex and age of the child or children involved
      ■ whether one child featured more regularly than others
      ■ what activity was taking place when an accident happened
      ■ whether the accident resulted in medical treatment.
   b) Consider whether the information tells you anything significant. Are there any obvious patterns or is the information random?
   c) Check the accidents that occurred against the risk factors on page 7.
2 What do you think are the most hazardous areas and situations you have found in doing this study?
3 Are the parents/carers routinely informed following an accident? If so, by what method e.g. in writing, by telephone or verbally on collection of their child? Is there a policy for this or is it an informal procedure?
4 Could any of these accidents have been prevented?

Accident information

Accident data and information is collected from a variety of sources, both statutory and voluntary. Individual government departments collect and analyse data for their own areas of responsibility.

The exact numbers of injuries and deaths from accidents varies from year to year, but differences between the major types of accidents show little change.

The demands on the National Health Service due to accidents are considerable, both in time and expertise of staff and in the costs. However, the greatest toll is upon the child and her carers.

Accidental injuries in and around the home

The United Kingdom, under the Department of Trade and Industry (DTI) has two continuous monitoring systems of accidents: the Home Accident Surveillance System (HASS) which monitors home accidents in the home and garden, and the Leisure Accident Surveillance System (LASS) which monitors outdoor accidents, away from the home. This information is collected from patients and staff at Accident and Emergency departments of eighteen large hospitals and used as a basis to estimate the numbers and types of accidents nationally.

Injury numbers, however, do not always give the most accurate information. The definition on an 'injury' may vary and some minor incidents will be treated and managed at home and so are never recorded. The injuries recorded on the DTI monitoring system do not include children seen and treated by their local general practitioner.

Fatal injuries

The Office for National Statistics (ONS) collates information on fatal accidents (deaths) from the coroners' returns in England and Wales. In Scotland and Northern Ireland this data is produced from the area Registrar General.

Road deaths and injuries

The Department of the Environment, Transport and the Regions (DETR) collects, analyses and collates information on road deaths and injuries.

STATISTICAL ANALYSIS OF DATA

Statistical information from all sources is used to:
- determine areas of concern
- identify the full nature of hazards and start necessary action
- inform the public and professional bodies about safety facts
- detect areas needing additional research
- stimulate preventive campaigns and raise public awareness
- influence product standards and design
- provide current accurate statistical information that is used by interested groups.

These statistics can help child care settings to:
- find out which situations and places are the most hazardous and likely to cause accidents
- plan safely using proven facts
- prioritise the types and amount of safety equipment to buy and maintain
- decide the type of staff training needed
- influence professional practice.

The above sources tell us that in 1997 in the UK:
- 459 children under fourteen years died from accidents

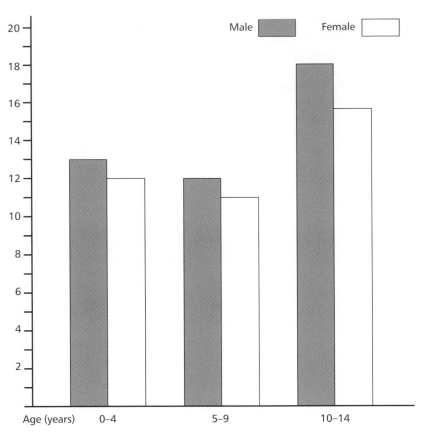

(NB These percentages, estimated from HASS 1997, do not always sum to 100 due to the effects of rounding)

Boys consistently have more accidents than girls

- one child in every four, roughly 6,500 per day, or 2.4 million annually, attended an Accident and Emergency department of a hospital following an accident
- children from social class V are five times more likely to die from accidents than those in social class 1
- boys consistently have more accidents than girls (see page 10).
- one in six of all children in hospital is there because of a possibly preventable accident.

Accidental injury in and around the home, nursery and school

The place where a child spends most of her time is where she is at greatest risk of injury or death.

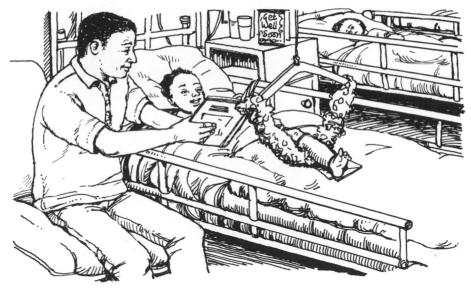

One in six of all children in hospital is there because of a possibly preventable accident

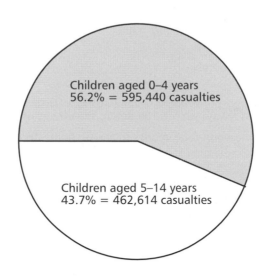

Children aged 0–4 years
56.2% = 595,440 casualties

Children aged 5–14 years
43.7% = 462,614 casualties

(NB These percentages, estimated from HASS 1997,
do not always sum to 100 due to the effects of rounding)

Accidents (non-fatal injuries) in the home to children aged 0–4 and 5–14 years

HOME INJURIES

The following statistics relate to non-fatal injuries in and around the home and include the garage, garden and garden equipment. The majority of injuries

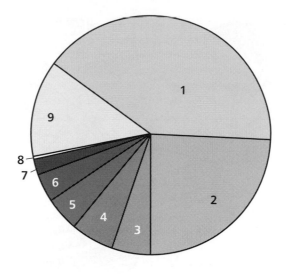

1 Falls 40.5%
2 Injuries associated with throwing or being hit by objects 24.3%
3 Cuts and puncture injuries 5.2%
4 Injuries involving foreign bodies 5.8%
5 The effects of heat and/or cold, burns and scalds 4.6%
6 Suspected poisoning 3.8%
7 Bites & stings 2.1%
8 Suffocation 0.4%
9 Other 12.9%

(NB These percentages, estimated from HASS 1997,
do not always sum to 100 due to the effects of rounding)

The most common non-fatal injuries following home accidents for all children under 15 years

happen in the living room where a child spends most time. However, the kitchen is the room where the most serious accidents take place, especially for a child under five. In 1997, out of a total of 67,000 injuries to children following accidents in the kitchen, 45,000 of these casualties were to children under five.

Falls
Falls account for approximately 40.5 per cent of all home injuries to children under fifteen. Most are caused by tripping or stumbling, but falls on stairs are particularly significant for children under five. The most serious falls are from windows and balconies and falls between two levels onto hard surfaces.

Injuries associated with throwing or being hit by objects
Injuries associated with throwing or being hit by objects account for 24.3 per cent of all home accidents. The majority happen from children running into

objects. However, injuries caused by thrown missiles are significant in boys over five. Boys are more at risk than girls.

Cuts and puncture injuries
Cuts and puncture injuries account for 5.2 per cent of all home injuries. The causes are various, ranging from everyday activities such as handling cutlery and using tools incorrectly to injuries resulting from the increased use of glass in the home.

Injuries involving foreign bodies
Injuries involving foreign bodies account for 5.8 per cent of all home injuries. They range in severity and include beads pushed up noses etc.

The effects of heat and/or cold, burns and scalds
The effects of heat and/or cold, burns and scalds account for 4.6 per cent of all home injuries. Fire and scald injuries are often serious and result in fatalities (see page 17).

House fires involving children are often associated with children playing with matches and lighters, chip pan fires and faulty wiring.

Scalding by the spilling of hot drinks is also significant.

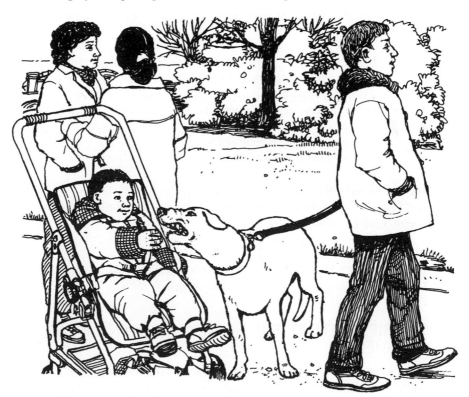

A toddler learns by exploration – some dogs are unused to children

Suspected poisoning

Suspected poisoning accounts for 3.8 per cent of all home injuries. A wide range of poisons is involved including family medicines, especially iron tablets, household chemicals, plants, cosmetics, alcohol and cigarettes.

Bites and stings

Bites and stings account for 2.1 per cent of home injuries.

Suffocation and choking

Suffocation and choking account for 0.4 per cent of all home injuries. They include choking on small toys, peanuts and other food.

Other injuries

Other injuries account for 12.9 per cent of all home injuries and include a variety of injuries that cover several categories or other less common injuries such as the effects of radiation and chemicals, and extreme over exertion.

Accident information also demonstrates that certain types of home accidents occur more frequently in children of different ages (see page 15).

INJURIES IN DAY CARE AND SCHOOL SETTINGS

Crèche or nursery

For 1997, LASS figures estimate that a total of 7,017 children under five attended hospital following injury in a crèche or nursery. Of these:

- 946 children were under one year
- 1,695 children were aged two years
- 2,405 children were aged three years
- 1,636 children were aged four years
- 335 children were aged five years.

Injuries in school

For 1997, LASS figures estimate that 15,019 children under eight years attended hospital following injuries in school.

Injury in school playground

For 1997, LASS figures estimate that 40,661 children under eight years attended hospital following injury in school playgrounds.

INJURIES OUTSIDE THE HOME (EXCLUDING ROAD CRASHES)

LASS statistics cover data collected from accidents in public areas, including parks, playgrounds, swimming pools, shopping areas and the open countryside.

For 1997, the national estimate for children under fifteen years attending

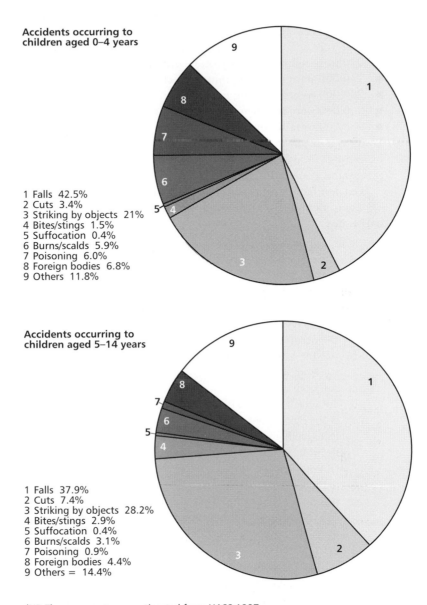

Accidents occurring to children aged 0–4 years

1 Falls 42.5%
2 Cuts 3.4%
3 Striking by objects 21%
4 Bites/stings 1.5%
5 Suffocation 0.4%
6 Burns/scalds 5.9%
7 Poisoning 6.0%
8 Foreign bodies 6.8%
9 Others 11.8%

Accidents occurring to children aged 5–14 years

1 Falls 37.9%
2 Cuts 7.4%
3 Striking by objects 28.2%
4 Bites/stings 2.9%
5 Suffocation 0.4%
6 Burns/scalds 3.1%
7 Poisoning 0.9%
8 Foreign bodies 4.4%
9 Others = 14.4%

(NB These percentages, estimated from HASS 1997,
do not always sum to 100 due to the effects of rounding)

The types of injuries in the home vary according to a child's age

Accident and Emergency departments following injuries outside the home was 1.3 million. Among these:

- 230 were as a result of near-drowning incidents from pools and open water
- 270 were following injury on farms and farm land
- 150,000 were following injury in school and public playgrounds
- 200,000 were following garden injuries
- 200,000 were following injuries in parks or public gardens
- 250,000 were following sport activities, the majority from football injuries.

Water is a major hazard for young children, they can drown or injure themselves in minutes in as little as three centimetres of water. More children drown in the ponds and pools belonging to their neighbours than in their own gardens.

Garden hazards include tools such as forks, spades, rakes and shears, electrical equipment such as mowers and hedge trimmers as well as chemicals and barbecues.

Activities

1 Assess local playground safety. Visit your local children's playground and assess the following.
   a) Where is it situated in relation to busy main roads? How easy and safe is the access?
   b) Are the external boundaries intact and secure to prevent young children running out?
   c) Are dogs excluded?
   d) For which ages of children do you consider the playground is designed?
   e) Is the equipment, (climbing frames, swings etc.) in good, safe, condition? Is it stable and secure? Is it well sited or, for example, can children be easily hit by swings?
   e) Of what are the surfaces of the playground made?
   f) Is there litter or debris around?
   g) Is the playground supervised and, if so, at what times of the day?
   h) Are children using the playground, if so, are they playing purposefully using the equipment correctly?
   i) Are children of different ages using the frames and swings at the same time with potential for danger? Are any older children obviously in charge of young children?
   j) Is there a supervisor? Does he or she intervene if the equipment is used in an unsafe way?

2 In addition, find out which department of the local authority is responsible for playgrounds.

3 Write a report on your findings and include a plan of the playground. Comment on any unsafe features that you feel should be changed. Remember, photographs are helpful to illustrate physical worries over a particular aspect of the ground. You may find the short section on community playgrounds (chapter 5, page 133) helpful for this activity.

FATAL INJURIES (DEATHS) FOLLOWING ACCIDENTAL INJURIES

Fatal injuries have declined in the last forty years. However, the numbers remain significant and in 1997, according to the ONS, the number of children under fifteen years who died in the home and on the roads was 459 – approximately nine children every week. Of these deaths, 301 were boys and 158 girls.

Fire is the major cause of fatal accidents in the home. In 1997, in the UK, according to Home Office Fire Statistics, 78 children under sixteen died due to fire. Of these 78 children:

- 5 children were under one year
- 33 children were aged one to four years
- 40 children were aged five to sixteen years.

Of the 78 children, 13 died from the direct result of burns, the remaining children from the effects of heat and fumes.

In 1997, in England and Wales, according to the ONS, the major causes of death excluding road traffic fatalities were:

- fire and flames: 40 children
- suffocation: 33 children
- drowning: 31 children
- falls: 21 children
- inhalation and ingestion including food: 18 children
- accidental poisoning: 4 children.

KEY POINT

Road deaths form the largest number of fatalities.

Accidents on the road

Children over the age of five are more at risk of death or injury on the road than from any other cause. However, even though traffic has increased, child fatalities have not risen with it. The United Kingdom has one of the lowest child death from a road accident rates in the world. Children under fifteen are 20 per cent of the population in the UK but account for only 14 per cent of the casualties and 7 per cent of the fatalities.

In 1997, according to the DETR, of children under fifteen years involved in road accidents:

- 255 were killed
- 6,197 were seriously injured
- 38,092 were slightly injured.

IN BUILT-UP AREAS

Of the 36,956 child casualties in built-up areas that happened in 1997:

- 49 per cent were pedestrians

- 20 per cent were cyclists
- 26 per cent were car occupants.

IN NON-BUILT-UP ROADS

Of the far fewer 7,588 child casualties in 1997:
- 82 per cent were car occupants
- 6 per cent were pedestrians
- 6 per cent were cyclists.

KEY POINTS

- Of all casualties, half were car occupants.
- Approximately two thirds of all child road accident casualties occurred on built-up roads.
- In recent years, fifty times more children have been killed from being run over while playing in the streets than have been killed by strangers (*Children's Play Council*, Tim Gill, 1999).
- Road accidents are the greatest cause of death in children over five years.

FACTORS WHICH INFLUENCE ROAD CASUALTIES IN CHILDREN

Speed is the main factor affecting death rates – the faster the car the more serious any resulting accident. If a pedestrian is hit by a driver travelling at 40 mph there is a nine out of ten chance of death, but if the car is travelling at only 20 mph then the chance of death is reduced to one in ten. It is estimated that seven out of ten drivers regularly break the speed limit in a 30 mph area with serious consequences to child pedestrians. Even 5 mph above the limit means the extra stopping distance is about six and a half metres.

Other influences that increase accident likelihood include children living on dense housing estates with many parked cars obstructing clear views for both drivers and pedestrians. Busy main roads with difficult crossing places, especially if only intermittently supervised by lollipop patrols, are also hazardous.

Poverty, overcrowded and poorly designed housing estates with no safe designated play areas often result in children playing in the street. Children living in such homes are particularly vulnerable to road and other accidents.

Children are at increased risk on the roads as they get older and the casualty rate is highest for children at primary school. Thirty per cent of child pedestrian accidents happen when children are going to and from school. Accident numbers are greatest between 7 and 9 am and between 3 and 6 pm.

The effects of accidents

The effects of any accident (see page 20) will, inevitably, depend on the severity and circumstances of how and when it occurred. The biggest single cause of

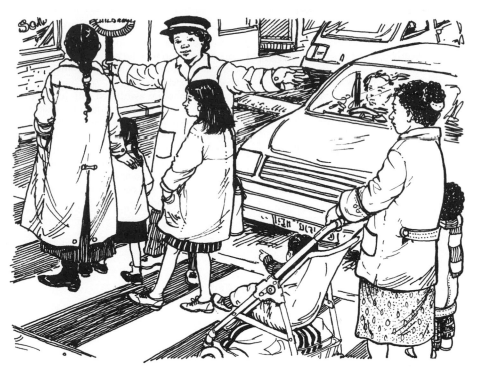

Always use supervised crossing points when available

accidents is human error. Even if an incident is minor, parents and carers should use the situation constructively to reassess child care management and routines.

THE EFFECTS OF ACCIDENTS ON THE FAMILY, CARERS AND SOCIETY

Emotional and social effects can be significant and wide ranging, especially if a child is badly hurt. Parents and carers, inevitably, feel responsible if their child has an accident whilst in their care and feelings of worry, guilt and shame are common, made worse if the accident was caused by adult negligence. As well as the care and attention needed by the victim, parents and carers, too, will need understanding and support following an accident.

Unresolved guilt feelings can have long-term effects, occasionally resulting in the affected child being over protected. This may lead to other children within the family having inappropriate restrictions placed upon them as parents worry about their safety.

Siblings may feel rejected, anxious and worried. An accident and Emergency department can be frightening for a child accompanying a sibling to hospital. The staff and family may be so involved in coping with the emergency that the sibling's needs may be overlooked, increasing that anxiety and fear.

Possible physical effects

Pain: short-term and long-term
Scarring, especially if associated
with burns and scalds
Longer term disability
Plasters and slings impeding
movement
Frustration associated with
immobilisation
Interruption in physical skill
development
Muscle wastage

Possible social and emotional effects

Loss of confidence in own ability
Loss of desire to try new activities/learn new skills
Increase of minor ailments e.g. tummy aches,
headaches, sickness
Occasional phobias associated with source of accident
Poor perception of body image in the child over five,
made worse if accompanied by scarring
General regression in behaviour including:
- bed wetting with associated embarrassment
- less ability to separate from parents/carers
- crying easily for no apparent cause
- being socially less confident with peers
- sleep disturbance

ON CHILD

Possible effects of hospitalisation

Time away from nursery/school
Break in learning/consequences for progress
Separation from parent/carers
Separation from siblings
Interruption in the development of social relationships, especially
in a school-age child
Boredom
Negative image of health personnel if associated with painful
procedures

General effects

Legal implications for the institution where the accident occurred
Effects on the relationships between parents/carers and child care
workers
Increased anxiety levels in staff/feelings of guilt and personal
responsibility
Negative effects on the careers of carers
Reassessment of accident procedures and practice, improved
commitment to staff training.

Possible effects of an accident

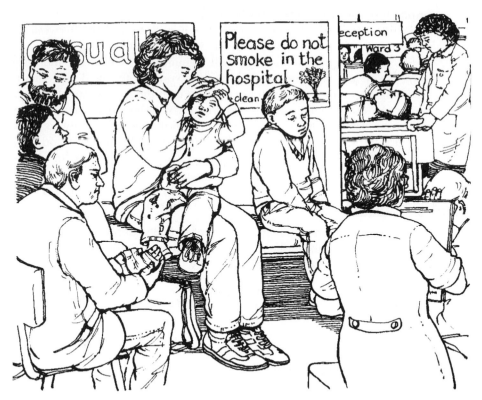

Siblings can feel neglected and become anxious in hospital

Financial effects

The financial burden on the National Health Service due to accidents is difficult to measure accurately, but is thought to be in the region of £300 million annually. This figure is for immediate emergency treatment and does not take into account accidents that may result in prolonged hospital admissions and repeated surgery (for example, skin grafts needed for children with burns or scalds). The result is that large sums of money are spent treating accident victims and this means that financial resources are diverted from other services.

For the family, financial loss may occur if repeated hospital visits are required. Long, expensive journeys may mean a parent or carer has to take time off work to accompany a child to hospital appointments resulting in losses in salary and extra travelling expenses.

Long-term implications

Following a very serious accident a child's long-term future might need major changes. She may need to go to a school nearer home, she may be restricted as to the activities she can join in, especially sport, and even some future career hopes may no longer be realistic.

Implications for the professional worker

You will, inevitably, feel guilty and worried if an accident happens while a child is in your care. Your own reputation may be affected if you are seen to have been careless or lacking in sound judgement. Families may feel anger and resentment towards you and may lose trust and faith in your professional judgement. These reactions can occur even if you are faultless or if the facts are unclear. Strain and worry can occasionally cause parents to verbally lash out when they see their child is in pain and danger, and in the heat of the moment apportion blame that may not be warranted. You must remain calm and in control and, if you are working in a team, seek support and advice from senior staff members (see 'The responsibilities of professional workers', page 180).

REMEMBER

Even apparently minor accidents can disrupt a child's confidence and security. Peers who may have seen the incident can also be affected. Consider how you can adapt your practice to promote emotional recovery.

HOW YOU CAN HELP THE CHILD AND PROMOTE RECOVERY

- Understand that her normal behaviour may be temporarily changed.
- If she wants to talk about her accident, be available to listen.
- Answer her questions honestly and give age-appropriate explanations.
- Offer opportunities to draw and paint if she cannot express verbally how she feels.
- Offer her activities to soothe her tensions such as dough or water activities.
- If she is displaying aggressive behaviour, channel this with physical activities such as running, jumping, shouting, banging drums.
- Use stories and rhymes and music for distraction.
- The older child might like to act out anxieties and fantasy in role play with friends.

KEY POINT

Be sensitive to her as an individual – children respond differently to difficult situations.

Safety influences

In addition to the child care worker and all adults and children with whom she comes into contact, other groups and agencies have important roles to play in child safety.

- Law enforcement agencies ensure safety regulations are kept, and mount prosecutions if laws are broken.
- Politicians, as policy makers, monitor and legislate for a safer world.

- Television and newspaper journalists report facts and provide articles and information on topics of immediate interest.
- Voluntary bodies have expertise and knowledge of a variety of safety topics. They frequently provide funding for research and produce information on safety facts and topics and run safety awareness campaigns.

Potentially large numbers of people and groups have both influence and interest.

Those mainly in informal roles or in group situations include:
- parents and siblings
- nursery nurses
- childminders
- teachers
- health visitors
- environmental health officers
- general practitioners
- architects
- the Police
- health promotion officers
- the media e.g. television.

Those mainly involved in the monitoring of standards and the environment include:
- local authorities
- health authorities
- education departments
- British Standard Trading Institute
- home safety officers
- trading standard officers
- The Health and Safety Executive.

Those mainly involved in research, information and raising public awareness include:
- charities such as the Child Accident Prevention Trust and The Royal Society for the Prevention of Accidents
- The Department of Trade and Industry
- publishers and the media in providing videos, books and magazines
- television and radio companies.

REMEMBER

Many of these agencies will have overlapping roles.

KEY POINTS

- Parliament is responsible for the framing of safety legislation.
- Manufacturers have a legal responsibility to produce safe goods, toys and equipment (see chapter 4).

Activity

1 Television is highly influential in many lives and can be effective in addressing popular issues of concern. Watch an episode of a current soap opera on television.
   a) Look at the way children and their care are portrayed.
   b) Do you consider the children's needs are represented realistically?
   c) What safety messages, either positive or negative, did you receive from the episode?
2 Discuss your findings with your peer group.

QUICK CHECKS

1 What is the most dangerous place for a child under five?
2 Where is the most dangerous place for a child over five?
3 Why is a sound knowledge of child development important in the prevention of accidents?
4 What are the dangers of over protecting a child?
5 How can you boost a child's confidence to learn skills to increase her safety?
6 What factors from a child's home life may increase the chances of an accident?
7 What social factors increase the chances of an accident happening?
8 What do you understand by the term 'role model' and what is its importance in child accident prevention?
9 How can we use accident statistics?
10 How many children a year die from accidents at home and on the roads?
11 What are the most common types of accidents for all children under fifteen?
12 What is the most common cause of accidental death?
13 How many children, is it estimated, will attend an Accident and Emergency department annually, following an accident?
14 Who are most vulnerable to accidents, boys or girls?
15 Why do you think children under five are particularly vulnerable to poisoning?
16 Which type of garden ponds cause most drowning accidents in children?
17 What is the most important factor affecting death rates in road accidents?
18 At what times of the day are children most at risk of injury on the road?
19 Name five possible social and emotional effects a child may have after an accident?
20 Give one example for each of the following:
   a) an informal safety influence
   b) an agency involved in safety monitoring.
   c) a charity concerned with child safety.

2 HEALTH AND SAFETY AT WORK

This chapter covers:
- Legislation
- Policies, procedures and risk assessment
- COSHH and RIDDOR
- Emergency procedures
- Premises and space standards; staff:child ratios
- Equipment: safety standards and safety marks
- Legal implications of accidents

Carers have a legal and moral duty to provide children with a safe environment. Good child care practice incorporates accident prevention and maintenance of good health, through working to high safety standards, as well as the ability to deal with accidents and emergencies if and when they occur.

Legislation

Much current safety legislation is initiated by European Union (EU) directives which establish a common standard throughout the Union. However, the laws covering the subject of the directives, are drafted and implemented by individual EU countries.

Legislation in the UK relating to the health and safety of children, within which all care and education settings must work, includes:

- The Health and Safety at Work Act 1974 (HASAWA) and Management of Health and Safety at Work Regulations 1992
- The Children Act 1989, in particular, Guidance and Regulations Volume 2, Family Support, Day Care and Educational Provision for Young Children 1991
- The Food Safety Act 1990 and The Food Safety (General Food Hygiene) Regulations 1995.

Regulations are often produced in order to clarify or elaborate on a certain part of an Act or to satisfy an EU directive. They have the same legal force as their parent Act.

Approved Codes of Practice (ACOPS) and Guidelines are not law, but are an official interpretation of the law. They set out standards of good practice which you should follow, so demonstrating you are complying with the law. For example, The Health and Safety Executive produces ACOPS and Guidance Notes to complement The Health and Safety at Work Act and its subsidiary Regulations. The Department of Health produces Guidance and Regulations to

The Children Act which incorporates both regulations and guidance on their interpretation.

THE HEALTH AND SAFETY AT WORK ACT (HASAWA) 1974

The Health and Safety at Work Act 1974 is the primary statute covering health and safety at work in the United Kingdom. This Act contains the principles for the protection of employees and any other persons who might be affected by the activities of a particular setting.

The HASAW Act and Regulations require that all settings have safety policies and working procedures that, 'so far as is reasonably practicable', avoid or reduce the risk of accident or injury. A competent person (or persons) must be nominated to manage Health and Safety. Employers with five or more employees must have a *written* Health and Safety policy.

THE CHILDREN ACT 1989

The Children Act 1989 and its Regulations place duties and responsibilities on local social services departments and education authorities with regard to the health, safety and welfare of children under eight years of age in a range of day care and education settings and enables them to impose such reasonable requirements as they consider appropriate in each case. This may include the writing of a Health and Safety policy, irrespective of numbers of employees, and conducting risk assessments.

Day care and education provision for the under eights includes:
- day nurseries
- playgroups
- childminders
- carer/toddler groups
- pre-schools
- nursery schools and classes, primary schools
- after-school clubs
- holiday playschemes.

As part of their duty to protect children, local authorities are currently responsible for maintaining registers of nurseries, pre-schools, childminders and playgroups. On-going registration is subject to a satisfactory annual inspection of care, education, hygiene and safety practice, carried out by individual authorities. This procedure is currently under review with the greater involvement of Ofsted anticipated.

REMEMBER

As demanded by HASAWA, and reinforced in The Children Act, nurseries and other day care centres and schools must ensure no harm comes to the children entrusted to their care, to the staff (employees), or to parents, carers, inspectors, tradespersons and other visitors to the setting.

THE FOOD SAFETY ACT 1990 AND FOOD SAFETY (GENERAL FOOD HYGIENE) REGULATIONS 1995

The Food Safety Act and Regulations set standards for making sure that food supplies for human consumption are pure and wholesome. It is against the law to sell contaminated, inferior or incorrectly labelled food, or to mislead the consumer with incorrect advertising.

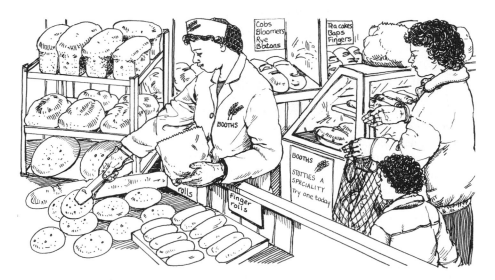

Good food hygiene practice – protective clothing, hair covered, gloves, bread tongs

Legislation and good practice must be followed by all those handling and preparing food in a variety of premises including day care settings and schools. Environmental Health Officers (EHOs) are responsible for enforcing the law and have a right of inspection of such premises and powers to close down any found to be unsuitable and unhygienic. Short courses in food hygiene and good practice, leading to a basic Food Hygiene Certificate, are widely available. Nursery and school managers should ensure food handlers in their settings are suitably trained.

Strict rules apply to personal hygiene before and during the preparation of food, cleaning and use of kitchen utensils, washing up and food disposal (see chapter 6, page 163). Food hygiene and the prevention of food poisoning is covered in greater detail in chapter 6, page 160.

A Government-appointed Food Standards Agency to monitor food safety on behalf of the consumer is to be introduced shortly.

Policies, procedures and risk assessment

Without clearly stated policies and procedures there would be muddle and lack of direction in the workplace leading to indecisiveness, too many inadequate 'personal' procedures (resulting in a higher risk environment) and a greater number of accidents.

The current philosophy on safety is based on risk assessment. A risk assessment is a careful examination of what, in your workplace, could cause harm to the children, staff or visitors so that you can develop safe working procedures and take precautions to prevent this harm.

Training all members of staff in the same safe procedures and working to a safe pattern demonstrates a professional attitude and sense of responsibility.

POLICIES AND PROCEDURES

A policy is a statement of intent about how management will act in the future and how they will address and act on all relevant issues. In this instance, the subject is child health and safety and a policy will state how management will establish good practice in that area. (Child Protection policies and procedures are set out in chapter 7.)

A Health and Safety policy
A Health and Safety policy contains three parts.
- A *statement* of commitment to safety is signed and dated by a governor, owner or senior manager.
- The *organisation* for implementing the policy names the person in overall charge of Health and Safety and others who are responsible for particular aspects of Health and Safety concerning the setting.
- *Arrangements* set out the procedures for safe practice, that is, physical checks on the setting plus details of how all routines and activities are carried out to ensure good overall Health and Safety practice.

REMEMBER

The workplace Health and Safety policy should be given to staff to read at the beginning of their employment and when it is updated. It must be available to parents on request.

An example of the first part of a Health and Safety policy for a day nursery – Part I, The Statement of policy – is given on page 29 and an example of the second part – Part II, Organisation – is given on page 30. Part III, Arrangements (see page 31) must be tailored to suit individual settings and will depend on the number of children, the ages of the children, the type of building and the local environment. Part III Arrangements can be written using the other chapters in this book as a menu to select appropriate Health and Safety practices.

XYZ NURSERY HEALTH & SAFETY POLICY

PART I   Statement of policy

a) The prevention of accidents and ill health to the children and staff of this nursery and to anyone who visits the nursery is of paramount importance.

b) Health and Safety matters are some of the most important considerations for our manager.

c) The setting will develop an organisation with clearly defined responsibilities for implementing and monitoring the policy.

d) Sufficient resources will be allocated to enable the policy to function effectively.

e) All identified risks will be eliminated or reduced as far as possible by:

- introducing a planned and systematic approach to all our activities
- the careful selection of safe equipment and materials
- the maintenance of a healthy and safe environment
- the use of physical controls (stair gates, window locks, non-slip floor coverings etc.) and by safe systems of work, for example, closely supervising children on steps and stairs and climbing equipment and teaching them how to use them safely
- careful selection of competent staff.

f) Information, instruction and training will be provided to all staff to enable them to develop and maintain a culture of health and safety awareness.

g) The Health and Safety practice of the setting will be monitored and the policy reviewed periodically.

h) Competent persons will be invited to provide assistance on Health and Safety matters, for example the Fire Prevention Officer, Environmental Health Officer, Day Care Adviser, Health Visitor.

i) The policy will be made available to the local authority, staff and parents for their inspection.

j) The policy will be revised and updated as and when necessary.

Signed......................   Date..............

Name.......................

Position.....................

An example of Part I, the Statement of policy, in a Health and Safety policy

XYZ NURSERY HEALTH & SAFETY POLICY

PART II   Organisation

Our nursery has a manager with three senior members of staff each in charge of one of the three different age groups. Each senior has a number of assistants.

The Manager

Responsibility for the implementation, operation and performance of the Health and Safety management system lies with the manager. Help will be provided, if required, to review and develop the policy, provide information on current and new legislation, and provide guidance on hazard identification and risk assessment.

The manager must be broadly familiar with the legal requirements for Health and Safety in the setting (local authority requirements, HASWA Regulations) and with the Health and Safety management system of the setting. He/she will set a personal example in all Health and Safety matters and ensure:

a) the safety of the setting is monitored and any shortcomings remedied
b) interest and enthusiasm for Health and Safety is promoted in the setting
c) sufficient resources are allocated to ensure the Health and Safety policy is implemented
d) all members of staff are adequately trained in Health and Safety matters
e) adequate supervision is maintained in all departments
f) all members of staff are aware of their responsibilities as laid down in this policy
g) all accidents and incidents are dealt with in an appropriate way
h) all staff know, and are practised in, their particular responsibilities in emergencies
i) all new staff are made aware of the Health and Safety issues in the setting and are shown how to work safely
j) sufficient and suitable safety notices, appliances and First Aid facilities are provided
k) access of visitors, including parents, is monitored and controlled.

Senior Staff

Senior members of staff have specific Health and Safety responsibilities, both in their own departments and for their assistants.

They will:

a) have a reasonable knowledge of the Health and Safety requirements for their position
b) organise their departments to ensure minimum risk to the children and staff
c) carry out daily safety checks in their nursery departments e.g. toys, equipment and materials, lavatory/hand washing areas and outdoor play areas
d) ensure the staff are familiar with their duties, including emergencies
e) set a personal example in Health and Safety matters
f) report all accidents and incidents to the manager
g) report any hazardous and unsafe conditions to the manager.

Junior Staff

Will have a reasonable knowledge of their responsibilities for Health and Safety in the setting and:

a) be aware of their roles in emergencies
b) carry out their work in a healthy and safe manner
c) report all accidents and incidents to the senior member of staff.

An example of Part II, the Organisation, in a Health and Safety policy

Part III, Arrangements includes how you are going to promote good practice in:

- personal presentation of members of staff e.g. dress code, permissible jewellery, storage of personal belongings, smoking policy
- familiarisation with emergency exits, positioning of fire extinguishers and smoke alarms, access to First Aid equipment and the evacuation of the setting in an emergency such as a fire
- conducting regular indoor and outdoor safety checks on the premises and equipment
- maintaining a clean and hygienic environment, including adequate ventilation, daily cleaning routines, cleaning up body fluids
- storage of cleaning materials
- wearing protective clothing
- caring for children at arrival and departure times
- supervising feeds, food preparation and mealtime routines including the setting's rules about nuts, especially peanuts

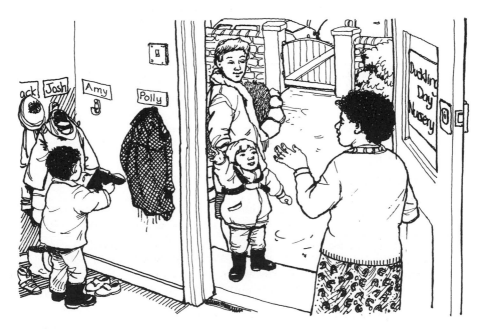

An adult known to the staff collects a child

- carrying out children's personal care routines such as nappy changing, toileting and hand washing
- organising and supervising play routines and outings
- lifting and carrying babies and young children to avoid harm to the child or carer
- dealing with and reporting emergencies such as accidents
- care of a sick child and administering medicines
- excluding children and staff with an infection.

RISK ASSESSMENT

The aim of risk assessment is to make sure that no one in the workplace gets hurt or becomes ill. It must show that 'suitable and sufficient' consideration has been given to the risks in the setting and adequate measures taken to prevent accidents or illness. Records should be kept to show proper checks have been made and precautions taken.

A risk assessment will ensure a safe environment and correct procedures. It should be:

■ carried out, initially, when a setting opens
■ reviewed regularly (perhaps once a year)
■ revised whenever circumstances require it – for example, when a new baby or toddler unit is opened, or a department is expanding to care for children with special needs.

Local authority social services and environmental health departments can advise on risk assessment.

KEY POINT

Risk assessments will vary in content according to particular work setting requirements. However, the following five trigger words are common to all risk assessments: **hazards, risks, controls, monitoring, review**.

There are five steps to consider in any risk assessment.

Step 1 Identify hazards

A *hazard* is something with the potential to cause harm and includes poor child care practices.

a) Walk around the setting, indoors and outdoors, and identify the hazards, for example stairs, electrical sockets, radiators, garden ponds, poisonous plants, animal fouling.
b) Consider an outing and identify the hazards, for example traffic, strangers, uneven pavements, animals, water.
c) Think about feeding babies and identify the hazards, for example milk too hot, contaminated milk.

Step 2 Assess risks

A *risk* is the likelihood of the hazard causing harm. Based on the hazards identified in Step 1 decide who might be harmed and how the harm can occur, as in the following examples.

a) Children indoors and outdoors at the setting: could they stick fingers and objects into electrical sockets, receive burns from radiators, fall into a garden pond, eat poisonous plants or contact a disease from animal faeces? Children, staff, parents, visitors: could they fall on the stairs?
b) Children on an outing: could they be struck by traffic, approached by a stranger, bitten by an animal, trip up on a pavement, nearly drown or be involved in a drowning accident?

c) Babies: could they receive a scald injury from hot milk or water or an infection from a contaminated feed?

Step 3 Implement controls

A *control* is a measure to eliminate or reduce a risk. Evaluate the risks in Step 2 and decide whether existing controls and precautions are adequate, or if more should be done to control the risk, as in the following examples.

- Are there gates at the bottom and top of the stairs? If not, are they necessary? Are stair coverings non-slip and in good repair? Is there adequate lighting on the stairs?
- Are electrical points accessible to children? If yes, are socket covers in place?
- Can the temperature of the radiators be safely regulated? If not, can thermostatic controls be installed?
- Is the garden pond covered with rigid netting or fenced off? If not, can this be done or should the pond be filled in? Filling in the pond eliminates the risk, netting or fencing only protects against the risk.
- Are the poisonous plants accessible to the children? If yes, remove them.
- Is the sand pit covered when not in use? Are fences and gates in good repair? Are loose-fill safety surfaces raked daily? Are animals kept out of the garden? If this is not possible devise a procedure for checking the outside area daily before the children go out to play (especially on a Monday morning) and remove any animal fouling.
- Is the staff:child ratio adequate to protect children against the above assessed risks during an outing? How do you decide on appropriate venues?
- Are the procedures for sterilising babies' feeding bottles and teats and preparing feeds adequate? If not, what steps are you going to take to improve them?
- What procedure is in place for testing the temperature of babies' feeds?

The risks remaining after implementation of these controls are known as 'residual risks' and should be examined to see if they can be further reduced or eliminated, as in the following examples.

- Although you will be fitting stair gates there is still the risk they may be left open. How will you control this residual risk? You may need to consider a regular checking procedure and further staff reminders and training, or fit automatic closures. Gates with alarms which sound when a gate is left open are available.
- The radiator thermostatic controls could fail causing overheating. This residual risk, which could cause a burn injury, can be eliminated by boxing in, or putting guards around, the radiators.

Step 4 Monitoring

Make sure you have a *monitoring* system to ensure the controls are implemented and maintained, as in the following examples.

- Are there regular safety inspection routines of stair gates, radiator temperatures, radiator guards, pond fencing, outside gates and perimeter fencing etc?

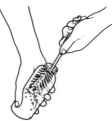

1 Wash the bottles, teats and other equipment in hot water and detergent. Use a bottle brush for the inside of bottles. **Do not rub salt on the teats.** Squeeze boiled water through the teats.

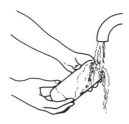

2 Rinse everything thoroughly in clean running water.

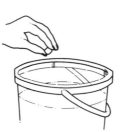

3 Fill the steriliser with clean, cold water. Add chemical solution. If in tablet form, allow to dissolve.

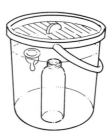

4 Put the bottles, teats and other equipment (nothing metal) into the water. Ensure everything is covered completely by the water, with no bubbles. If necessary, weight down. Leave for the required time according to manufacturer's instructions.

The correct procedure for chemical sterilisation of feeding equipment

- Are outings planned efficiently with correct staff:child ratio? Are checks done to evaluate the plans for an outing? (See chapter 3, page 70.)
- Is hygiene practice in the milk kitchen or food preparation area adequate? Do you check the procedures for sterilisation of feeding equipment, making up feeds and temperature testing (see page 35) are carried out correctly?

Step 5 Review
Review your risk assessment as and when previously suggested (see page 32).

KEY POINTS

- At the end of any risk assessment, check that you have complied with all the local authority safety regulations and standards and that you have a written record of the assessment.
- Safety in the setting should be on the agenda of every staff meeting.

1 Check that the formula has not passed its sell-by date. Read the instructions on the tin. Ensure the tin has been kept in a cool, dry cupboard.

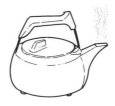

2 Boil some **fresh** water and allow to cool.

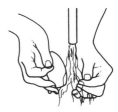

3 Wash hands and nails thoroughly.

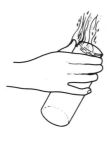

4 Take required equipment from sterilising tank and rinse with cool, boiled water.

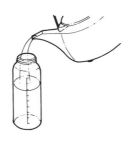

5 Fill bottle, or a jug if making a large quantity, to the required level with water.

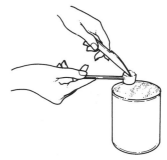

6 Measure the **exact** amount of powder using the scoop provided. Level with a knife. **Do not pack down.**

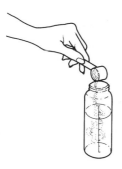

7 Add the powder to the measured water in the bottle or jug.

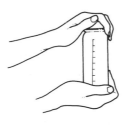

8 Screw cap on bottle and shake, or mix well in the jug and pour into sterilised bottles.

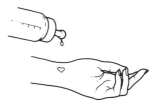

9 If not using immediately, **cool quickly** and store in the fridge. If using immediately, test temperature on the inside of your wrist.

Correct procedures for preparing a bottle feed and testing the temperature of the feed

COSHH and RIDDOR

The Control of Substances Hazardous to Health (COSHH) and the Reporting of Injuries, Diseases and Dangerous Occurrences Regulations (RIDDOR) are two important supplementary Regulations introduced under HASAWA 1974.

COSHH

The COSHH Regulations 1999 help to protect people in the workplace against health risks from certain substances. Health problems from a variety of substances can include:

■ skin irritation, dermatitis and skin cancer from handling harmful substances
■ burns and injuries to hands and eyes from contact with corrosive liquids
■ asthma and other lung conditions due to inhalation of toxic (poisonous) and irritating substances
■ poisoning from ingesting toxic liquids.

KEY POINT

Allergic skin and respiratory conditions from using latex rubber gloves are currently causing concern. The gloves are used by staff in many day care settings when carrying out nappy changing routines and dealing with body fluids. Allergic reactions, which may be mild or more serious, can be prevented or reduced by the use of powder-free or synthetic gloves, though both are more expensive.

A system of labelling dangerous substances (see page 37) indicates the risks from using them. Information on labels and safety data sheets, giving additional information, should be requested from the supplier to enable substances to be used safely. Substances used for cleaning and maintaining the setting need to be assessed together with those used in schools for science, art and craft, design and technology (CDT) activities.

A register of materials used on the premises should provide information about the hazards they present, how they should be used and details of First Aid procedures if there is an accident with them.

Domestic bleach is likely to be the most common hazardous substance used in a nursery (see page 38). Bleach is often used to disinfect lavatories and floors, but it gives off fumes which can irritate the eyes and lungs of both children and staff. Fumes also form if bleach and lavatory cleaners are used together or mixed with

Symbol	Classification	Symbol	Classification
	Flammable		Toxic
	Corrosive		Harmful
	Explosive		Irritant

These COSHH symbols are black on an orange-yellow background.

Supply labelling required by UK legislation

urine in the lavatory. Make sure the lavatory windows are open when you are using bleach and that you flush a lavatory containing bleach or cleaner before any child uses it.

Whatever substance you are using (bleach, lavatory cleaner, sterilising agents, disinfectants and so on) always read the manufacturer's instructions regarding handling, dilution and use.

REMEMBER

Although substances carrying a COSHH label are the most dangerous and must be stored in a safe, secure place where no child can reach them, all substances and cleaning materials in your setting must be carefully used and kept in a separate locked cupboard.

WARNING
- Thick Bleach.
- Contains Sodium Hydroxide.
- Contains Sodium Hypochlorite.
- Irritating to eyes and skin.
- Avoid skin and eye contact.
- Keep out of reach of children.
- Warning! Do not use with other products. May release dangerous gases (Chlorine).

IRRITANT

FIRST AID:
If swallowed, seek medical advice immediately and show this container or label. In case of contact with eyes, rinse immediately with plenty of water and seek medical advice.

A sample label from a container of domestic bleach

Activity

Look around your work setting.

a) Check for, and list, substances with a COSHH symbol. Household bleach and correction fluid are likely to be on your list, but there may be others such as insect repellent and caustic soda. Some glues used in creative activities may also carry the symbol. Check the symbols on the containers against the symbols on page 37 so that you understand their meaning.

b) Where is bleach stored in your workplace? What is the recommended dilution of the bleach?

RIDDOR

The Reporting of Injuries, Diseases and Dangerous Occurrences Regulations (RIDDOR) 1995, requires certain accidents, injuries and illnesses to be reported to the enforcing authority – for schools and day care settings this means the local authority. Reporting procedures are as follows.

- Deaths, and any injuries which require a child, parent or visitor to be taken from the setting to hospital, must be reported immediately (by telephone) to the local authority.

- The local authority must be notified on form F2508 if members of staff sustain injury, or become ill, *as a result of their work* and are subsequently absent for more than three days, but death or serious injury must be reported immediately by telephone

Serious injuries and reportable diseases are listed in RIDDOR Regulations, but if in any doubt contact your local authority for advice.

All accidents and incidents, however trivial they may appear, should be recorded in an accident book.

Emergency procedures

Evacuation of children and staff from your workplace may be necessary because of a fire, bomb or gas alert or other serious incident. To minimise and control such an incident make sure:

- written notices (in different languages) for evacuation of the premises are displayed in the entrance hall, in every room and next to every telephone in the setting. Notices must be clearly visible to staff, parents and visitors. When necessary, the information must also be available on tape, in large print or in Braille
- all emergency exits are signed with a mandatory green and white 'running man' pictogram, the arrow indicating the direction of the exit. Two examples are shown on page 40. Make sure you know where these exits are, and at all times that they are unlocked, free from obstruction, and can be opened easily from the inside. It is illegal just to have a sign with words such as 'Emergency Exit'.
- there are designated outdoor assembly points and systems for clearing the building and accounting for all children, staff, and any visitors on the premises. All staff must be aware of these procedures and their role in an emergency.

FIRE PREVENTION AND PROTECTION

Currently, nurseries, playgroups, childminders and schools are not required to hold a Fire Certificate. However, local authorities make fire safety precautions a condition of registration for day care facilities and childminders. Schools should have written regulations covering fire prevention and emergency evacuation procedures, approved by the governors. Local fire prevention officers will visit day care and education premises at the request of the local authority and advise on fire safety. Recommendations and advice given by an officer should be implemented. This may include:

- changing some materials used for, or on, walls
- changing some items of furniture
- the number and location of fire extinguishers
- fitting 'linked' smoke alarms (able to be heard in all parts of the building). Alarm sensors should not be located in kitchens, bathrooms or garages where fumes or steam can trigger the alarm
- siting of fire doors and emergency exits (they must open in the direction of escape)
- staff training in fire practice procedures, including raising the alarm, use of fire extinguishers and evacuation of the premises.

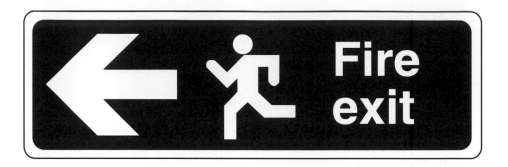

Fire exit

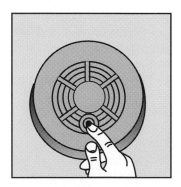

Smoke alarm BS5446

Two examples of acceptable Emergency Exit symbols, plus a smoke alarm BS5446

KEY POINTS

- Fire extinguishers must be regularly checked (at least annually) by the Fire Officer or approved firm.
- Check smoke alarms weekly, keep them clean and dust free.
- Install a fire blanket in every kitchen.
- Make sure an emergency lighting system is available.

Fire prevention

Fire is a major cause of accidental death. Fire prevention is a major part of safe practice. To reduce the means of initiating fire in the setting:

- consider your smoking policy. Preferably, there should be no smoking allowed on the premises. If smoking is allowed, there should be a designated 'smokers room'
- make sure there are no naked flames except in the kitchen. Keep children out of the kitchen
- obtain a certificate for the electric wiring in the building
- ensure electrical appliances and systems (including computer suites) are well maintained and checked regularly by a competent person.
- check that there are no frayed or trailing flexes, and no overloaded sockets
- fit covers on sockets when not in use
- check that curtains and furnishings are non-flammable
- use appropriate fireguards for all heat sources
- reduce the amount of combustible materials e.g. stored or used paper from drawing and painting activities.

Fire alarms and fire practice

A recognised alarm system e.g. a fire bell or electronic alarm, plus smoke and heat detectors and alarms, has to be in place, maintained in working order and regularly tested. A whistle is not considered an appropriate alarm as children become accustomed to the sound of a whistle during PE and other activities.

Each setting must have its own written fire practice procedures stating individual departmental and staff responsibilities. New staff must be trained in emergency procedures on joining the setting.

The procedures should be practised at least every term to familiarise staff (including part-time staff) with them and ensure the children can be evacuated quickly and safely. Try to vary the scenario by pretending an emergency exit is blocked off or a room is filled with smoke.

KEY POINTS

- There are no rules as to whether fire practices should be announced or initiated without prior warning. The most important factor is that staff are trained in how to respond to a fire emergency – an unannounced fire practice is of little value if staff are untrained.
- The best protection for children and staff in the event of a fire is to give early warning and evacuate via a safe route to a safe place.

Knowing the policies and procedures of the setting and your own role and responsibilities is an important part of teamwork and safe practice, enabling you to respond in a calm, efficient and prompt manner to an emergency.

Always keep a record of every fire practice, and evaluate your practice and procedures.

Activity

Find out from the local Fire Prevention Officer, or different voluntary organisations, what adaptations to the environment and alarm systems are necessary for evacuating children with:
- visual impairment
- hearing impairment
- mobility disabilities.

In the event of fire

In the event of fire you should know:
- how to raise the alarm
- who is responsible for contacting the emergency services (dialling 999)
- how the children are to be evacuated, how many babies or children can be carried by each member of staff
- which evacuation route is to be used by each room or department.

You should also know who is responsible for:
- checking specific areas (such as the lavatories) for remaining children; reassuring and taking care of shy and 'settling in' children; helping children with special needs and those for whom English is not their first language
- checking the registers at the assembly points
- declaring the building empty.

Once the alarm sounds the setting must be evacuated safely and quickly and the emergency services called. These two activities should be done simultaneously. Confirmation that evacuation is complete and everyone accounted for is essential. Always await clearance from the emergency services or senior member of staff before re-entering the building.

Activity

1 Read the fire notices displayed around your setting.
2 Check that you know where the emergency exits are in your setting.
3 If there was a genuine fire emergency in your workplace today would you:
    a) recognise the sound of the fire alarm?
    b) know your role in evacuating the children?
    c) know the designated assembly point?
    d) know how to use a fire extinguisher/fire blanket?
If your answer to any or all of these is 'no', then familiarise yourself with the correct answer/procedure as soon as possible.

Should a fire occur, you may have many children to look after outdoors (perhaps in the rain and cold), without their parents, for possibly several hours. Thought should be given as to how best to care for them – perhaps there can be an arrangement with a local school, community centre or church hall to use their facilities in such circumstances.

An up-to-date and accurate record of parents' home and workplace telephone numbers must be kept in case of fire or other emergency.

Premises and space standards; staff: child ratios

In accordance with The Children Act 1989, providers of day care and education services for the under fives are required to follow particular guidance for premises and space standards and staff: child ratios (see page 44).

PREMISES AND SPACE STANDARDS

The way that nursery space is used will vary but the following considerations should be common to all settings.

- No room, regardless of size, should have to accommodate more than 26 children except for special occasions. Where possible, the maximum number should be lower for younger children.
- A separate room for babies and toddlers with proper facilities both for preparation of feeds and for nappy changing close by must be provided.
- Laundry facilities with a washing machine and drier must be provided if very young babies are being cared for.
- Appropriate facilities for children with special needs must be provided.
- A minimum of one lavatory and one hand wash basin for every ten children must be provided. Wash basins must have hot and cold running water – hot water temperature at around 39°C (102 °F).
- For staff, separate toilet facilities, office space and a staff room must be provided.
- A kitchen of an appropriate size equipped to provide meals and snacks for children and staff should conform to environmental Health and Food Safety Regulations.
- An outside play space, preferably adjacent to the building and exclusively for the use of the children, should be provided. If this is not possible, proper arrangements must be made for the children to be taken regularly to local parks or playgrounds

Fixtures such as cupboards should be excluded when working out adequate space.

Desirable space standards in a day nursery

Age of child	Square feet	Square metres
0 to 2 years	40	3.7
2 to 3 years	30	2.8
3 to 4 years	25	2.3

Reproduced by kind permission of The Stationery Office, from *The Children Act 1989, Guidance and Regulations Volume 2* Seventh Impression, 1998

STAFF: CHILD RATIOS

Staff:child ratios in full day care settings may need to be higher than the standard recommendation in the table if:

■ not all the staff are qualified or suitably trained

■ you are caring for children with special needs

■ you are caring for babies under one year who need constant attention.

Standard recommended staff:child ratios for the under fives in day care and education settings

Type of setting/Age range	Ratio	Comments
Under 5 years' full day care 0 to 2 years 2 to 3 years 3 to 5 years	 1:3 1:4 1:8	Because of management and administration duties, managers or officers-in-charge should not be included in these ratios where more than 20 children are being cared for
Nursery schools and Nursery classes	2:20 (minimum)	One adult should be a qualified teacher and one a qualified nursery assistant
Reception classes in primary schools		Where 4-year-olds are attending reception classes in primary schools, the staffing levels should be determined by the schools and local education authorities
Childminding Under 5 years 5 to 7 years Under 8 (no more than three being under 5) years	 1:3 1:6 1:6	All these ratios include the childminder's own children and apply to nannies employed by more than two sets of parents to look after their children
Day care services for school age children Where 5- and 7-year olds are cared for on a daily or sessional basis (i.e. care at the end of the school day and full care in school holidays) Where facilities are used by children aged over 8 years as well as under 8 years	 1:8	A higher ratio may be necessary if children with special needs are being cared for. A lower ratio may be appropriate for some short sessional facilities not lasting the full day Providers should ensure that there are sufficient staff in total to maintain the 1:8 ratio for the under eights.

Reproduced by kind permission of The Stationery Office, from *The Children Act 1989, Guidance and Regulations Volume 2* Seventh Impression, 1998

Equipment: safety standards and safety marks

The major factor affecting the choice of nursery and school furniture, toys and indoor and outdoor equipment is safety, and the potential risk of injury or accident from individual items.

SAFETY STANDARDS

Accident risks can be minimised by buying products made to a recognised standard of design, quality, safety and efficiency and which carry a British (BS) or European (EN) number. With the emergence of the single European Market an increasing number of British Standards have become harmonised with their European equivalents. For example, BSEN 1466 (1988) indicates an agreed British and European Standard for carry cots (see table on page 46).

All products bearing a BS number are subject to testing by the British Standards Institution (BSI) or other testing organisation.

REMEMBER

Standards are re-written from time to time as specifications are up-dated. The table on page 46, 'Nursery Equipment – British and European Safety Standards', identifies five items of nursery equipment and gives the current BS and/or EN number together with the Standard specifications.

THE CE MARK

	The CE Mark	The CE Mark is a claim by the manufacturer that the product meets a British or European Standard of quality and safety although it is not a mark of approval by any official organisation. Products marked CE are entitled to free passage throughout the European Union

Nursery equipment – British and European Safety Standards

Equipment/ Safety Number	Standard specifications
Stair gate/ barrier (for up to 2 years) BS 4125 (1991) Available to fit stairs, windows, patio doors and for use as room dividers. Some have two-way opening	Non-toxic materials and finishes: will not harm child if sucked or chewed Locking device: cannot be unfastened or jerked free by a young child Width between vertical bars: 25–100mm (a new European Standard reducing this maximum width to 65mm, is proposed. Some stair gates are already available with gaps of 65mm) No features which could be used as playthings; no edges or points to trap fingers or flesh or cause other injuries Instructions provided for correct and safe assembly
Cot mattresses BS 1877 Part 10 (1997)	A 'safety label' stating size of cot for which the mattress is manufactured Gap around the mattress no bigger than 3–4cm at the top, bottom or sides to prevent a baby's head or limb becoming trapped Maximum depth: 100mm at edge; 150mm at centre Firm; cover fits exactly; of permeable material Fillings: safe and clean Fixed ventilators (if fitted) must not be positioned on the sleeping surface of mattress
Carry cots BSEN 1466 (1998)	Carry cot and stand: sturdy and stable when assembled, will not collapse when placed on slight slope or when baby wriggles or leans to one side No wheels or castors fitted A 'safety label' stating 'product is suitable for a baby who cannot sit up by itself, roll over or push up on hands and knees. Maximum weight of child 9kg' Fixed anchor points for safety harness Non-toxic material and finishes
High chairs BS5799 (1986)	Strong and stable: for children of 6 months to 3 years Raises child to height of dining table Child cannot slip between seat and tray nor be trapped in any way Smooth edges and corners, no fixtures or crevices to trap fingers or flesh or cause abrasions Fixed anchor points for safety harness Integral crotch strap
Dummies/Soothers BS5239 (1988)	Made from safe, non-toxic material Teat is smooth and free from flaws, does not easily disintegrate Has passed tests for bite resistance Carries instructions for sterilising and storing

SAFETY MARKS

A Safety Mark indicates that a product is type approved for safety. The table below lists particular Safety Marks which you need to be able to recognise and understand.

Safety Marks

Mark	Name	Meaning
	BSI Kitemark	Indicates a product has met a British safety standard and has been independently tested
	Lion Mark	Indicates adherence to the British Toy and Hobby Association Code of Practice and ensures a product is safe and conforms to all relevant safety information
	Age Warning pictogram	Indicates: 'Warning – do not give the toy to children less than 3 years, nor allow them to play with it' Details of the hazard e.g. small parts, will be near the symbol or with the instructions
	BEAB Mark of the British Electrotechnical Approvals Board	Indicates that electrical appliances carrying this mark meet a national safety standard
	BSI Safety Mark on gas appliances, light fittings and power tools	Indicates the product has been made and tested to a specific safety standard in accordance with the British Standards Institute
	Safety Mark on upholstered furniture	Indicates upholstery materials and fillings have passed the furniture cigarette and match tests – a lighted cigarette or match applied to the material will not cause the article to burst into flames
	Low Flammability labels	Children's pyjamas, bathrobes made from 100% Terry towelling and clothes for babies up to 3 months old must carry a label showing whether or not the garment has passed the Low Flammability Test. Either of these two labels is acceptable. Always look for these labels when choosing such garments.
	Keep Away From Fire label	Indicates the garment is not slow burning and has probably not passed the Low Flammability Test. Great care must be taken anywhere near a fire or flame

Children's nightdresses, nightshirts, dressing gowns and bathrobes (except 100% terry towelling bathrobes) **must** all pass a test for slow burning, so these garments do not need an additional **low flammability** label and generally do not carry one.

Activities

1 Visit the reference department of a main library. Ask for assistance in researching the British or British/European Standards for cots and playpens. For both items find out:

   a) the BS or BSEN number and the year of the Standard

   b) the main safety specifications.

2 Write up your findings and discuss them with your college tutor and student

Legal implications of accidents

In the event of an accident, the setting could be prosecuted under criminal law for breach of statutory regulations. It could also be subject to a claim for damages under civil law. So, if a child or employee is seriously injured, and if the injury has been caused by a failure to comply with statutory regulations, a nursery or school could be prosecuted by the local authority Health and Safety Officer or, in the case of a fatality, by the Crown Prosecution Service. The setting could be fined or custodial sentences could be imposed on the owners or managers.

KEY POINT

No insurance can be taken out to ensure against any costs or fines involved in a criminal prosecution.

A civil suit can be pursued by an injured child's parents or carers to compensate for the hurt, trauma and possible cost of long-term care. This could result in a very large award against the setting, possibly running into hundreds of thousands of pounds. Although insurance should pay for this cost, insurance premiums will increase dramatically.

If an accident was found to be the result of negligence or a lack of proper safe procedures in the setting, the setting may be judged by the local authority to be unsuitable for the care and education of young children and its registration withdrawn. Even if registration is not withdrawn, parents are unlikely to entrust their children to the setting.

QUICK CHECKS

1 Which organisation initiates much current safety regulation?

2 Which three Acts of Parliament are referred to in this chapter?

3 What do you understand by a 'policy'?

4 When is it compulsory to have a written Health and Safety policy?

5 What are the three important components of a Health and Safety policy?

6 What do you understand by 'risk assessment'?

7 Following an initial risk assessment, when a child care setting newly opens, when might subsequent assessments be carried out?

8 What are the five 'trigger words' to remember when carrying out a risk assessment?

9 What does COSHH stand for?

10 List four health problems which can be caused by substances carrying the COSHH label.

11 Why is it important to flush a lavatory containing bleach or cleaner before a child uses it?

12 What does RIDDOR stand for?

13 Is there a legal requirement to comply with COSHH and RIDDOR Regulations?

14 In what emergency circumstances might it be necessary to evacuate a nursery or school?

15 Where in the setting should written notices for evacuation of the premises be displayed?

16 Describe the sign which must, by law, be displayed at all emergency exits.

17 What safety advice will the Fire Prevention Officer offer a nursery or school?

18 What fire prevention measures could you take in your work setting to reduce the possibility of a fire?

19 What do the following safety marks found on products tell you about those products? a) Kite Mark b) Age Warning pictogram c) Lion Mark d) BEAB label e) 'Keep Away From Fire' label.

20 What legal recourse do parents have if their child is seriously injured in the setting she attends?

3 CHILD DEVELOPMENT AND SAFETY

> ## This chapter covers:
> - **Babies**
> - **Toddlers**
> - **Early years: 3–5 years**
> - **Key stage 1: 5–7.11 years**
> - **Supervision of children in groups**
> - **Outings**

Understanding how a child thinks and develops enables you to plan safely. All children proceed through set stages of development but not always at the same time or rate. A knowledge of the range of normal development, will help you to decide if a toy or activity is suitable for a child's stage of progress and so allow you to plan for her safety needs. This is especially important when working with children with special needs and children who have been denied access to certain experiences.

REMEMBER

Cross check this chapter with the information in chapters 4 and 5.

Babies

THE DEVELOPMENT OF BABIES: BIRTH TO TWELVE MONTHS

A new-born baby	A new-born baby will: ■ have uncoordinated reflexive body movements ■ have limited head control ■ have large jerky movements of her limbs, especially her arms ■ cry to indicate distress.
At 3 months	At three months a baby will: ■ hold her head up whilst on her back and for a few seconds when held sitting ■ wave her arms symmetrically ■ kick vigorously ■ sag at her knees when held upright ■ when placed on her tummy, support herself by pushing on forearms ■ begin to watch her own fingers in play

- hold a rattle but will be unable control her hand movement
- by four to five months, begin to roll over
- suck well but will be unable to manage lumps
- enjoy being handled and care routines.

At 6 months

At six months a baby will:
- sit with support in a cot or pram, and for a few seconds will be able to sit unsupported on a firm surface
- move her arms purposefully
- bounce on her feet when held on a hard surface
- vocalise, laugh and scream to indicate emotion
- begin to locate sounds
- reach and grasps for toys – usually two handed – and enjoy manipulating toys
- transfer everything to her mouth
- begin to distinguish between strangers and known adults.

At 9 months

At nine months, a baby will:
- sit alone and unsupported for reasonable periods
- have sufficient balance to lean forward and pick up a toy
- be highly active, rolling, squirming and often crawling
- pull to stand but will be unable to voluntarily sit back – she will fall backwards with a bump
- reach and stretch eagerly for toys
- use a scissors grasp to pick up toys and an inferior pincer grasp for smaller toys,
- pick up tiny sweets,
- still take most things to her mouth
- find a toy that is temporarily and partially out of sight
- hold finger food, and chew
- want to feed herself
- imitate action
- need some support when sitting for dressing on an adult's knee
- understand 'no' and 'bye'
- vocalise, babble and enjoy attention.

At 12 months

At twelve months, a baby will:
- sit confidently and often stand unaided
- crawl or shuffle on her bottom and may crawl upstairs
- be efficient at getting around her own environment
- pull to stand and release voluntarily
- use furniture to support her around a room
- possibly walk, or maybe walk holding an adult's hand
- use a fine pincer grasp for picking up small objects
- use both hands freely
- hold an object in both hands simultaneously
- know her own name
- vocalise constantly
- begin to understand several words
- respond to simple instruction
- have acute hearing
- drink from a cup with help
- chew, but may find hard lumps difficult

- wish to be involved in mealtimes and will hold a spoon but will not be effective at getting it into her mouth
- continue to take most things to her mouth
- show affection.

IMPLICATIONS FOR SAFETY

A baby is totally dependent upon her carers. All accidents that happen to a pre-mobile child are the direct result of adults' actions or failure of the adult to anticipate the child's developmental progress. As a baby becomes more mobile, you must anticipate and eliminate potential dangers, yet still provide a learning environment. The changes in her development are rapid and sometimes unexpected.

Safety checks for the new-born baby
- Never leave an unguarded baby on a changing mat placed on a high surface.
- Pillows and duvets can cause overheating and possibly suffocation, so are unsafe.
- Plastic coverings for mattress must be tightly fixed and fitted otherwise they can loosen and smother a baby.
- Do position the baby on her back (supine) (see chapter 5, pages 125 and 126) preventing cot death.
- Check that any knitted clothes or shawls are tightly woven so they cannot catch small fingers and restrict blood supply.
- A dummy on a ribbon around her neck is dangerous. If one is needed, attach it with a safety pin to her clothes, if necessary with a cord or chain no longer than 20cm.
- Supervise babies in baths at all times.
- In the home, turn the hot water thermostat down to 54°C (129°F) to reduce the chances of scalding. Nursery temperatures may be lower, often 39°C (102°F) (see chapter 5, page 110).
- Never leave a baby unattended in public, even in her pram. Remember, a baby will go happily to any stranger in the first months of her life: this makes her vulnerable to snatching if not supervised.

Safety checks for the developing baby
- Always supervise her when bottle feeding. Leaving her with a bottle propped for her to manage herself is dangerous.
- Use fixed harnesses, with shoulder straps in high chairs.
- High chairs must be stable and broad based. Make sure that she cannot reach out and grab, or kick at, unsafe objects.
- Delay introducing weaning foods until at least four months, unless recommended, and only offer lumpy food when she can manage, usually not before seven months. Never add salt to any home-cooked foods given. Make bottle feeds up, hygienically and to the correct dilution (see chapter 4, page 91).
- Stay with her at mealtimes, never leaving her unattended, particularly with finger foods and when introducing food with lumps.

- Keep a baby, who is crawling, out of the kitchen and away from ovens, washing machines and tumble dryers – use a safety gate or playpen if necessary.

Safety checks for working with babies
- Keep a clutter free environment so you do not stumble and trip. Remove loose mats, and do not carry a baby on wet or slippery floors.
- Wear suitable shoes and lift carefully (see chapter 4, page 99).
- Never run when carrying a baby.
- When travelling in a car, transport her safely (see chapter 5 page 131).
- Never drink hot liquids with a baby on your lap or pass them over a sleeping child.
- Do not smoke whilst a baby is in your care.
- Use smoke alarms and check they are working and the batteries functioning.
- Use kettles with short, curly flexes when a baby is crawling or rolling. Keep them away, out of reach, at the back of the work surface.
- Check all safety equipment, especially fixed fireguards and plug sockets. Check that cooker or hob guards are in place, working and used at all times (see chapter 4, page 77).
- Check that furniture is stable, dangerous objects are out of reach and corners are protected, before a baby begins to pull herself to stand or cruise.
- Keep animals away from a baby. She will investigate dogs and cats the only way she knows, by poking and pulling at eyes and ears – they may respond by biting.
- Check that windows have security locks and have safety glass or are covered with safety film to prevent shattering.
- When working with more than one baby or with groups of children of mixed age range, maintain the recommended ratio of staff to children (see chapter 2, page 43).
- A new baby, whether a sibling or a baby fresh to a group, will cause interest and maybe jealousy to a toddler. He or she may try to examine the baby, for example, by poking her, trying to carry her or offering her toys that could be swallowed, so never leave younger children unattended with a baby.

Everything a baby has will be transferred to her mouth. This is a highly sensitive area where she learns the shape and texture of an object, so think about what she may reach for to put in her mouth. It might:
- be swallowed, for example calculator batteries, household medicines or small toys
- be inhaled directly into her lungs, for example peanuts
- obstruct her airway, for example plastic bags or balloons
- fragment and pieces may be torn off and inhaled, for example crumbly foods or cushion foam
- be toxic, for example paints, berries, house plants, alcohol or cosmetics.

KEY POINT

Always anticipate the next stage of the baby's development. Development can be rapid and unexpected, in fits and starts, and she may reach previously unsafe areas and objects before you realise she has the ability.

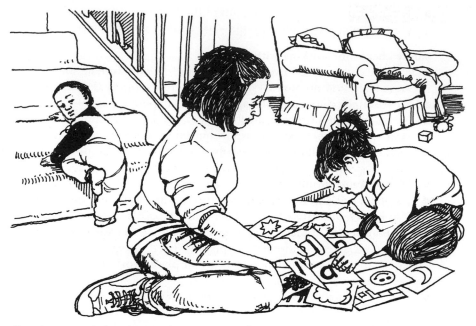

Developmental changes can be unexpected

Safety education for babies

Introduce the idea of hot, cold, sharp and so on, and say 'no' for dangerous areas, but use 'no' sparingly, saying the word quietly and firmly. Because she copies your 'no' or shakes her head, when she nears a fire, for example, this does not mean she will remember or transfer this information to another fire in a different room or understand that heat is retained even after the glow is gone. Similarly if you say 'no' to everything, her ability to learn about levels of danger will be lessened, together with the effectiveness of a 'no'. Adapt her environment to reduce risks and show her safe practice. She will enjoy imitating your actions and learn as a result. Sitting down when drinking, using implements correctly, handling animals gently – these all teach informally and effectively.

Baby walkers

While all carers are keen to promote mobility, there is no evidence that a baby walker will help. Opportunity to practise moving around firm furniture, keeping the child's feet bare to help grip and balance, and encouragement are the best ways to promote walking. Walkers teach a false sense of balance and may, in fact, cause delayed gross motor skills. They can promote a mistaken sense of security. It is often wrongly thought that if a baby is in a walker, she is safe, and as a result, doors are left open, stair gates not fixed and fires unguarded. Falling down stairs is the most common 'baby walker' accident. Health professionals and organisations such as the Child Accident Prevention Trust, the Royal Society for the Prevention of Accidents and the Chartered Society of Physiotherapy, do not recommend their use.

The responsibility for the child's safety is yours.

Activity

1 Create a treasure basket. This provides opportunities to promote sensory, physical and emotional development for a baby who is not yet crawling, but who sits steadily when unsupported. Fill a smooth, shallow, wicker basket with approximately ten to fifteen safe, stimulating, natural articles for the baby to observe, smell, feel and manipulate, listen to, and take to her mouth.
   a) What safety features must you consider when planning your basket?
   b) How would you test the safety of your basket and the contents?
   c) What non-intrusive supervision should you provide for the baby when she is given this basket?
2 Show your filled basket to your tutor, or placement supervisor, before offering it to a baby.

Toddlers

THE DEVELOPMENT OF TODDLERS

At 18 months   At eighteen months, a toddler will:
- walk well, stopping and starting confidently, occasionally keeping feet apart and arms out to help balance
- run, but will not always be able to avoid obstacles
- begin to walk upstairs, but will usually come down backwards or bump down
- push, pull and carry objects
- bend knees to pick things up from the floor, but use a hand to help regain balance
- finger feed herself
- use a spoon, but will often turn it over before it reaches her mouth
- use a cup to drink, but will need to use both hands
- use a delicate pincer grasp and is able to pick up and manipulate quite small objects such as beads and pins
- show preference for one hand, but will often use both at the same time
- continue, occasionally, to put objects into her mouth, but increasingly less often
- imitate adults' actions such as brushing her hair
- explore her environment insatiably
- use a range of words – usually about 20 to 30 words

- have quite a wide understanding of simple commands
- obey simple requests such as 'fetch your shoe, please'
- like her mother/prime carer in sight
- respond to ritual and routine but will get frustrated if thwarted, and possibly be distracted
- have good vision and hearing.

At 2 years

At two years, a toddler will:
- run, stop and start easily
- later in the year, walk up and downstairs confidently using a rail and two feet to a step
- push, pull and steer toys and large wheeled objects though not always avoiding obstacles, climb and push furniture to reach windows and other objects
- like to throw a ball but often will be unable to release it or judge where it is if she tries to kick it
- develop a sense of her own size in relation to areas, for example by fitting herself into cupboards when hiding
- have developing manipulative skills and will enjoy taking things apart
- pick up and replace small beads and other objects
- use a spoon to feed herself and be able to chew well
- remain very curious about her environment
- have little understanding of danger
- demand immediate gratification and be unable to wait for needs to be met –behaviour will be egocentric
- be unable to share and will vigorously defend toys, territory and her prime carer's time and attention
- enjoy make-believe play and this will develop meaningfully
- have increasing language skills and be able to make simple two or three word sentences
- by two and a half years, talk constantly to herself and others and be asking questions.

IMPLICATIONS FOR SAFETY

A toddler experiences wide developmental changes from life as a totally dependent baby to a child who is keen to explore and demonstrate her independence and developing skills. However, her skills are not always matched with power and control. If attending a day care setting, she will probably transfer to a room away from the babies where there is less close supervision. She is endlessly curious and inquisitive and has physical skills to reach a wider environment. She can now turn door handles to go outside, use furniture to climb to reach higher and further. She can manipulate objects, open drawers, unscrew bottles and so on. She is often unreasonable and egocentric. She has a limited under-standing of danger or the ability to wait for a dangerous situation to be altered. This, coupled with her desire for immediate gratification, makes it a hazardous age.

Safety checks for the toddler's environment
■ Make daily checks of her environment for hazards, especially if there are changes in routine, visitors, holidays, or other adults or children in the house.
■ Use safety glass in doors and windows. Windows that can be reached should have safety catches.
■ Use stair gates at the top and bottom of stairs, but teach her how to climb safely and come down backwards.
■ Organise your kitchen so that dangerous objects such as glasses, and plates and so on are inside high wall cupboards with locks if necessary. Place saucepans and durable cooking utensils lower down for her to explore.
■ Lock alcoholic drinks away in a cabinet.
■ Keep matches and cigarettes well away and out of reach.
■ Lock all medicines in a cabinet. If visitors are in the house, remind them that their medicines, including any vitamin and iron pills, must be inaccessible for a toddler. Always use child resistant tops but be aware that some children as young as three can open them.
■ Decide when she can be in the kitchen and use safety gates to exclude her when you are cooking or secure her in a high chair to watch you.
■ As a toddler enjoys hiding in small places, make sure she can get in and out of them, keep washing machines and tumbler dryer doors locked.
■ Ensure the front door does not have a handle she can reach and turn.
■ In the garden, supervise her at all times. Never leave her unattended near a paddling pool and remember that even a bucket of water or a puddle is potentially dangerous. Check that plants are non-toxic, the garden shed has a lock and outer gates and fences are secure.
■ Fence off permanent garden ponds and empty and upturn paddling pools and buckets after use.
■ Keep gardens clear of toxic chemicals and animal litter. Cover sand pits when not in use.
■ Check balcony safety (see chapter 4, page 82).
■ Check the safety of play areas in parks and playgrounds (see chapter 5, pages 132–135).

Safety checks for working with toddlers
■ Supervise meal and bath times carefully.
■ Distract her from forbidden objects, and be prepared for tantrums – she really cannot have something dangerous – but be calm and firm.
■ Plastic bags are not toys, so do not let her play with them or leave them around.

- Check that her clothing, including dressing-up costumes, cannot hinder her or trip her. Tie her shoe laces firmly, or use Velcro fasteners.
- Always consider toy suitability. Many toys, especially those with small parts, are not recommended for a child under three (see chapter 2, page 47). She will continue, occasionally, to put things into her mouth
- Look at toys for age recommendations and compare with her actual stage of development — too simple or too difficult will both cause frustration and mis-use with implications for safety. If she is tired, hungry or ill she may regress in behaviour and make some toys and activities she usually enjoys less safe.
- If you are working with children of mixed ages, remember that a child may have access to toys potentially dangerous for her developmental stage.
- Check the condition of equipment and toys daily, and wash these regularly (see chapter 5, page 116).

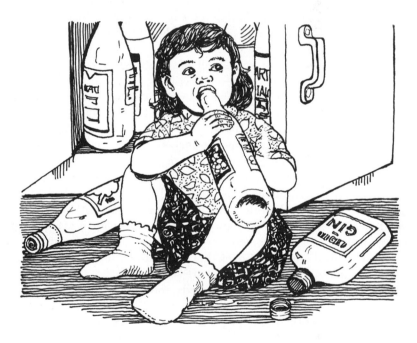

Young children cannot differentiate between the contents of bottles. Alcohol is poisonous to children.

REMEMBER

As the child's skills increase, think about what she might reach tomorrow. She will have surges in development. These are often linked with opportunity and developing confidence. She may learn to push a chair against a window, climb and reach for the catch in the space of a day, when previously she just climbed stairs.

KEY POINTS

■ When working with groups of children of mixed ages, some toys may be unsuitable for part of the group.
■ A toy may, in itself, be safe but how it is used may be dangerous.
■ Never leave a toddler unsupervised with a young baby.
■ For a child with developmental delay, toys with small pieces may be unsuitable for longer than expected.

Safety education for toddlers

Encourage the toddler to put her toys away when she has finished playing. Keeping a clutter free environment will reduce falls. Teach her to use equipment safely, show her how to handle her fork carefully, do not let her wave scissors or knives around or run while carrying potentially dangerous objects

Helping her up and down stairs safely will extend her skills. Try moving a stair gate one step higher at a time so she learns to climb gradually without the risk of falling down a flight. Encourage her to practise large motor movement safely: toddler gyms will help develop her strength, power and control, and she will have adult supervision and safety mats to cushion falls. Always explain why she needs to follow a certain action – she understands more than she can express. Remember that she finds waiting very hard, so only tell her what she cannot do in the present, not what will be forbidden tomorrow.

Take calm, firm stands about major safety issues, usually associated with roads and the outside world, for example holding hands along a pavement. Keep to these rules even if a tantrum is provoked, you must never compromise on safety issues.

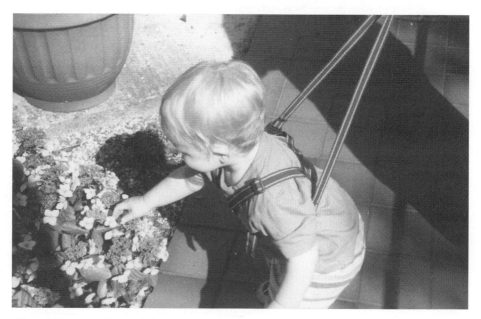

Allow him to explore safely

Check that you choose issues and say 'no' carefully and try to use compromise and distraction techniques at other times. For example, one small sweet given after a meal instead of a whole chocolate bar is a reasonable compromise, but allowing her to refuse to sit in her car seat is unacceptable at any time. If you can make her world safe by planning and anticipation, rules over major safety issues can be few and easily accepted. Do not leave, in her sight, exciting, forbidden objects that may be unsafe for her. Remember that her concentration span is limited and her recall of instructions will be affected by hunger, illness, tiredness, and excitement. Transfer of information from one situation to another is difficult for her.

KEY POINT

Encourage her to try new skills while you watch and reward with praise. The more opportunities to practise she has, in supervised situations, the safer she will be.

Activity
Children need to develop gross motor power and control to increase their safety and promote confidence, so, applying your knowledge of child development, arrange a suitable, safe and sturdy obstacle course for children aged between two and three years.
a) Provide large objects and equipment to let them: balance, slide, jump, roll, crawl, climb over and through and navigate and steer around.
b) Consider safety surfaces and the types of clothing they should wear.
c) What skills do you hope to extend?
d) What extra value is there if this course is outdoors?

Early years: 3–5 years

THE DEVELOPMENT OF THE EARLY YEARS: 3–5 YEARS

At 3–4 years	At three to four years, a child will:
	■ be skilled at walking up and downstairs
	■ climb, run and jump (with two feet)
	■ stand and walk on tip toe
	■ push, pull and manoeuvre large toys and objects
	■ ride a tricycle and pedal confidently
	■ thread beads and cut with scissors
	■ use a spoon and fork
	■ help in simple dressing and undressing, but not undo buttons or tie laces yet
	■ give her name and age
	■ enjoy using her developing language
	■ remain egocentric in many aspects of her behaviour, but

will share with her peers, although turn taking remains difficult
- have a developing attention span
- be able to listen to instructions, but to do this she has to stop any task in which she is involved
- begin to have an idea of basic time, for example yesterday, tomorrow or later
- have difficulty in understanding that things she watches on television may be unreal and she may try to copy actions she sees
- have a problem relating cause to effect – just because she does not want something to happen she thinks it will not.

At 4–5 years

At four to five years, a child will:
- be physically skilled, coming up and downstairs, climbing trees and ladders, riding and manoeuvring a tricycle
- have developing balance, and can stand, walk and run on tips toes and stand for several seconds on her preferred foot
- be able to throw, catch, bounce a ball and use a bat
- be skilful using a spoon and fork at meals
- dress and undress herself but will need help with laces and fastenings
- enjoy demonstrating her independence
- begin to manage to use words to explain frustrations and for solving arguments and quarrels
- be able to take turns
- continue to view the world essentially from her own point of view
- always question and ask constantly
- have speech that is recognisable by most adults, including strangers
- have an increasing attention span and can now understand instruction without breaking off from an activity.
- have an awareness that includes past, present and future.

IMPLICATIONS FOR SAFETY

As her independence increases she is keen to use her new skills. However, she does not always have total power and control over her movements to manage some activities competently and she may get frustrated if an adult attempts to take over. Her physical skills allow her to use playgrounds, parks, and outdoor areas more easily. Her manipulation allows her to open bottles and containers, even child-resistant caps, so offering challenges but also posing dangers.

Her understanding has now reached the sophisticated level of knowing something is there even when she cannot see it, so she is less easily distracted from dangerous but exciting situations, and she may remember to return later to the danger. She is also, possibly, less under the adult's eye than a child in a younger age group.

She is likely to be attending a pre-school group where she will need to follow instructions from adults other than her parents and carers. Her attention span is increasing, but she still can forget instructions if engrossed in an activity. She has a great respect for rules in games and can become distressed if these are changed, so a consistent approach from you is important.

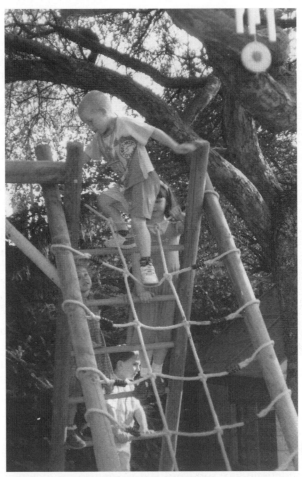

At four a child is skilled at climbing

Safety checks for the early years
Note: Some checks will be the same as the previous age ranges and the checks below should be linked to additional information in chapter 4

- Ensure you are providing opportunities for all-round skill development, including safe challenges, for example higher climbing frames, more objects to manipulate, fix and organise.
- Discuss safety rules and how to use equipment correctly and demonstrate, reinforce and check that the child has understood.
- Extend skills at mealtimes, offering knives to replace spoons, and as she becomes more competent, encouraging her to test the heat of her food.
- Organise her clothes to promote independence by offering her choices from a safe selection that will allow her to dress and undress easily. Floating dresses for use on climbing frames are obviously unsuitable but also remember to look at her footwear and check that it is non-slip, correctly fitting and with no laces that can easily come undone – Velcro fasteners are ideal.
- Consider that a toy or activity may be in itself safe, but only if used as directed. It may become unsafe when a group of children of different developmental stages are together. Also, toys may not always be put to the use for which they were designed – a bat can hit another child as easily as it hits a ball, but this does not make the bat itself unsafe.
- All outside play areas must be safe, equipment in good condition and external fences secure (see chapter 5, page 105).
- Decide on group safety rules, for example no running in the classroom, with food or with toys and tools. Explain why the rules are necessary clearly, and consistently monitor and reinforce these rules.

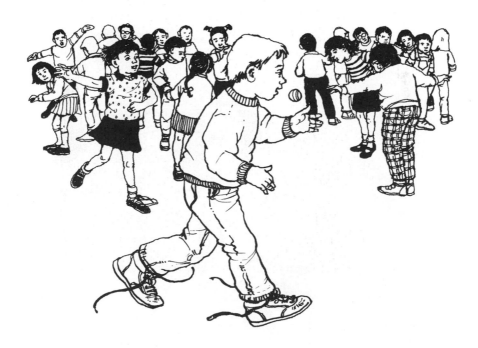

Check that shoes are suitable and that they fit. Also check that laces are tied

She is keen to learn and you must plan to extend her skills, helping her to climb higher, jump further, use a knife and cut with blunt-ended round scissors, all under supervision.

Safety education for the early years

Discuss safety ideas, and reinforce information with demonstrations showing and telling her how. A child of three and four will need repetition of instructions and rules. Always accompany these with explanations as to why she should follow a certain action or why something is not allowed – she is more likely, then, to comply. In praising her skill development you will increase her self-esteem and also her safety. If you stop her from experimenting and practising, within a supervised environment, she will become unsure and lack confidence and be more likely to make errors. If you do not like heights, are afraid of water and cannot swim, consider how you might be passing on non-verbal negative messages to a child.

Her language, by four, is clear and will allow her to get into conversations with other adults and now is the time to introduce the idea of strangers and how to respond to grown-ups not known to her. You must do this without making her shy and frightened of all adults – give her simple rules that are clear. Teach her name, address and telephone number to her, tell her to stay with the adult looking after her, not to go off on her own or with anyone else and to stay put if she gets separated on an outing. Teach her who are safe adults and include the Police in this list.

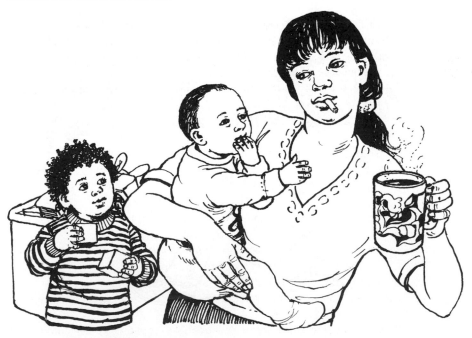

Remember, she learns by your example

A child of this age often enjoys swimming and has lessons at this age or younger. This is a valuable skill all children should have.

Teach her about roads, reinforcing the message that pavements are for people and roads are for cars. Explain and show her how you decide where to cross a road. Compare her height to a parked car, ask her if she can see over it, to reinforce a message that a car in the road would not see her either. Always repeat the stop, look, listen and think message. Explain to her about fast cars and slow people, hard machines and vulnerable children. Tell her parks and gardens, not roads, are for play.

Special ongoing thought and attention is needed for any child with a sensory impairment or developmental delay. Different safety instructions may be needed as she may not hear warnings, see obstacles, or be able to balance and control her movement effectively. She may also have difficulty in asking questions and understanding answers and any of these problems will be made worse in noisy group situations. Toys or activities may need adaptations for her particular need and any age recommendations on toys may be unsuitable.

KEY POINTS

- The child will continue to imitate your actions, so do not be tempted to behave rashly to save time or because you think you are not being noticed.
- Safety considerations must be integrated into all planning activities, routines and the curriculum.
- Up-date your knowledge of safety issues regularly.

Activities

1 Promote children's awareness of road hazards. Design a road circuit in your playground. Chalk in the junctions, make traffic lights and supply potential hazards. Provide bells and horns and use the wheeled toys available.
   a) Explain the functions of the red, amber and green traffic lights.
   b) Demonstrate the basic rules of stopping at junctions and looking and listening.
   c) Discuss road sounds and how cars and bicycles make themselves seen and heard.
   d) Introduce the idea of right and left and the way traffic goes.
   e) Use a stop watch to measure time taken for different types of wheeled toys to safely complete a circuit.
   f) Discuss the ideas of fast and slow, safe and unsafe.
   g) Ask the children to think about how they can be seen and heard on roads, and remember to include children with disabilities.
   h) Think of ways of involving the children in this activity, for example painting and making traffic lights, acting as lollipop people and policemen, saying and singing appropriate rhymes and songs.
2 How could this activity be adapted to meet the developing cognitive skills of children in Key Stage 1?
3 How could parents and carers be involved in reinforcing this learning in the real road and environment?

Key Stage 1: 5–7.11 years

THE DEVELOPMENT OF CHILDREN AT KEY STAGE 1: 5–7.11 YEARS

At 5–6.11 years   At this age, a child will:
- continue her rapid physical development
- now be jumping with a rope and starting to skip
- be able to ride a two-wheel bicycle with increasing control and balance
- have fine manipulative control to allow her to dress herself, begin to tie laces and manage small buttons
- at five and six, still have difficulty in relating cause to effect – she may not be able to predict the consequence of certain actions
- be keen to be independent
- be cross and frustrated if tasks are too difficult for her
- be reckless and enjoy challenges
- occasionally be quarrelsome with her friends but also need their approval
- have imaginative play which leads onto 'make-believe' games.

By 7–7.11 years   By this age, a child will:
- have more rational and logical thinking and this may include abstract thoughts
- begin to ask about cause and effect
- be able to begin to see someone else's viewpoint
- have increasingly sophisticated language.

By **eight years**, a child will be well on the road to reading.

IMPLICATIONS FOR SAFETY

It is only towards eight that a child begins to have some understanding that she has a role in her own personal safety. Up until this late stage, a child considers that things happen to her, not that she has a part in making a situation dangerous. This understanding is helped by her beginning to have abstract thoughts and ideas, so stimulate this area of her development.

Safety checks for 5–7.11 years
- Check general environmental safety as in the preceding check lists.
- Preparation and supervision of the potential hazardous activities she is now able to manage – cooking, bike riding, swimming – is important.
- Ensure she has the correct clothes and equipment for new activities – bright colours for walking and helmets for cycling. Remember, though, she is not yet ready for roads with her bike.

- Monitor peer pressure for dangerous challenges and be prepared to intervene.
- Be aware that bullying may develop within a peer group and be prepared to intervene.
- Understand that she will not be as rule bound as a nursery-aged child and may disobey safety instructions when with her friends. She will continue to need adult supervision.

Safety education for 5–7.11 years

Involve her and her peers in decision making and discussions over safety issues and rules. She is more likely to keep to rules if she is involved in their development. Discuss the dangers around her, how she can lessen them and why equipment must be used in certain ways.

Set physically demanding challenges at games times, it will release her excess tension and energy constructively, it will also help develop her skills and balance, and stimulate her judgement and reasoning. Ask for her cooperation in problem solving, perhaps by dividing her peers into groups to solve issues, for example discuss how to organise the gym equipment so she can reach the higher bar or how to make the most interesting assault circuit.

Continue to monitor consistently and reinforce group safety behaviour and rules.

Activity
Keep a safety log.
a) In the log or diary recording the work you plan and implement, list the unexpected safety issues that arise during your work.
b) Describe adaptations you need to make to activities you offer to children of different ages and group size.
c) Record the different levels of supervision that various activities require.
d) Record how often, and in what manner, you intervene in safety issues.
e) Do you think intervention would have been less with improved planning or anticipation?

Teaching road safety

GREEN CROSS CODE
Crossing a Road the Green Cross Code Way – Stop, Look and Listen:
1 Find a safe place to cross and stop.
2 Stand on the pavement near the kerb.
3 Look all around for traffic and listen.
4 If the traffic is coming, let it pass, look all around again.
5 When there is no traffic and the road is clear, walk straight across the road.
6 Keep looking and listening for traffic as you cross.

Many schools will have road safety teaching from professionals outside the school often involving the Green Cross Code. However, as formal road safety is linked to a child's individual experience and level of reasoning, it may not be effective for a child under eight years. She may not have the experience to implement the first instruction of the Green Cross Code to 'choose a safe place'

If other classroom-based teaching is given, the child may have difficulty in transferring the information to different and unexpected situations, becoming distracted and forgetful, so any formal teaching needs constant reinforcement. You can help by implementing the following actions.

- Increase her visibility with bright clothing, incorporating fluorescent material into jackets and using reflective, inexpensive, luminous bands over dark coats.
- Offer her experience on roads with you and show her your own safe actions.
- Discuss and plan road training for her own specific area and needs – her own route home, to school, playground or park.
- Raise her awareness of how quickly cars and bikes can travel.
- Always encourage walking, not running, telling her not to play with balls or toys when she is a pedestrian.
- Explain about unsafe crossings – the brow of a hill, corners of junctions, from behind a bus or car and when her sight is obscured.
- Encourage her always to use the inner side of the pavement, not to wait at the edge for a bus or car.
- Always encourage her to stop, look, listen and think when crossing roads with an adult.

Reinforce this teaching by the following actions.

- Help her find safe places to cross, especially if she is using busy streets with many parked cars, by choosing the largest gaps, easing out, and judging the distance.
- Involve her in decision making as to when it is safe to use a crossing.

KEY POINTS

- A child needs accompanying on most roads until she is ten or eleven, depending on her own individual personality, maturity and the area in which she lives.
- Bicycles are best used in parks and gardens for children under eight and many safety experts consider children should not ride on roads until they are eleven.

REMEMBER

A child who has a visual or hearing impairment will be especially vulnerable on roads.

Supervision of children in groups

Levels of supervision will vary according to the particular activity or routine taking place and the ages and abilities of the children involved. Supervision should allow and encourage a child to experiment, explore and achieve in safety. Children with special needs or developmental delay must be offered similar opportunities.

Make sure you always know who is in overall charge of a group of children and that there is a procedure for 'hand-over' to another member of staff. The children should be visible to staff at all times. The setting should maintain the correct staff:child ratios (see chapter 2, page 44).

An unsure, over-cautious and over-protective carer can leave a child feeling frustrated, angry and bored. This may lead a child to do something she knows is disallowed such as ill-using equipment or toys or becoming aggressive to other children. A tired carer can easily lose concentration and become less alert.

It may help to consider supervision under the following three headings.

GENERAL SUPERVISION

- During children's rest or sleep periods.
- Of older children during meals.
- Of older children during playtime.

CLOSE SUPERVISION

- Of babies and toddlers at all times, including mixed groups of toddlers and babies.
- Of children during cooking and woodwork activities.
- When children are playing on the climbing frame and other large structures. There should be rules in the setting about how many children are allowed on a particular piece of equipment at any one time.
- Of a child who feels unwell and is resting quietly.

CONSTANT SUPERVISION

- Of babies on changing mats.
- Of babies being fed.
- Of children in the bath or near water.
- Of children on outings, crossing roads and during swimming sessions.
- Of some children with special needs

Outings

Outings offer a child the experience of wider environments and increased learning opportunities. They may be informal – visits to shops and parks – or more structured outings for early years groups. All outings could, potentially, increase the risk of accidents because of:

■ changes in routine
■ excitement and possible tiredness in the children
■ lack of familiarity with the setting.

To lessen the chances of harm, careful organisation is needed.

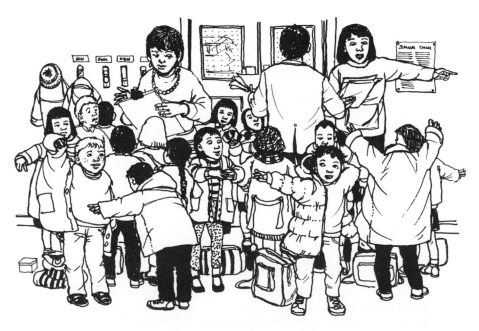

Changes in routine and excitement can increase the chances of accidents during outings. Planning and preparation are important

PLANNING

- Choose the destination and length of the outing to meet the age and developmental stage of the child or children. Aim to extend children's learning, by linking to current themes, topics or interest in the group. Ensure the outing is also fun for the children and involve them in the planning.
- Choose the time of year. Very cold, hot or wet weather for major outdoor outings may be unsuitable for toddlers.
- Pre-visit the venue, even if you have been recently, changes happen quickly that may affect the safety or pleasure of an outing. Confirm opening times, location of lavatories and toddler changing facilities, where lunches can be eaten and what shelter is available in hot weather or rain. Now, too, is the time to assess the physical environment for safety hazards, for example unfenced water, incomplete external barriers or overcrowding. If you have a child with a disability, check their needs can be met, for example that there is wheelchair access. Estimate travelling time and decide how the journey is best made, whether by car, bus, coach or foot.
- Ensure there is liaison between parents and carers. An exchange of information will be needed.

Liaison between parents/carers and the setting

A letter to the parents/carers outlining your proposed outing and its aims and objectives should be sent. The details you should give include:
- the duration of the outing with the estimated departure and arrival home times
- any cost
- information about food– whether a packed lunch may or may not be required
- advice that no glass bottles should be used
- suggestions as to suitable clothing and shoes including any necessary spares.

Ask parents/carers whether they would like to come. Many parents/carers like to join in outings and with sufficient notice can become additional accompanying adults.

From the parents/carers, you will need to obtain the following.
- Written consent to take the child out of the care setting.
- Details of any particular health problems relevant to the outing such as asthma, epilepsy, diabetes, allergies and intolerance. If the child requires medication ask that sufficient is brought with her. If the parent is not accompanying the outing, written authorisation to administer a medicine is necessary.
- Confirmation that parents'/carers' telephone numbers and contacts are accurate for the day.

Before the outing
- Decide on the ratio for accompanying adults. The following ratios usually apply:
  - children 0–2 years, 1 adult to 1 child

- Children 2–5 years, 1 adult to 2 children
- Children 5–8 years, 1 adult to 5 children.

If a child has a special need, for example behavioural or mobility difficulties, a one to one ratio whatever the age of the child may be required. Assess this on the child's particular needs. If the outing is long, or the journey complex, additional adults over the above ratio will be valuable.

- If you are using cars, or minibuses see chapter 5, page 129 for regulations covering transport and page 130 for seat belt requirements. If using buggies and prams, ensure they are in good condition with effective brakes and safety harnesses.

- Make a list of the children going on the outing and divide a large number into smaller groups with individual registers. State the times during the outing that children must be checked against this register. Allocate adults to the groups or individual children.

- Organise emergency back up – a child may be ill, a car break down or a train be cancelled. You will need a contact number and the name of the person available at the nursery, school or parent workplace. A mobile phone provides an efficient and easy means of communication.

- Decide what additional equipment you will need. Essential is a small travelling First Aid kit (see chapter 8, page 218). You may need sun hats, sun screen and extra clothing such as pants or nappies for toddlers. To support the learning aims of the outings you may need work sheets or bags to collect leaves, and so on.

- Make a timetable for the day and include your learning outcomes. Plan your follow up activities or associated work.

- Involve the children in discussing the outing and talk about what you will expect them to do. Explain basic safety rules and make your requests relevant to their level of understanding. They should be short and simple for the younger group. Wider considerations can be given to the older children, for example thought for their peers and the environment. Tell older children what to do if they become separated from their allocated adult and about keeping safe from strangers (see chapter 7, page 190).

- If visiting farms or zoos, explain to the children how to handle animals with care and sensitivity and when they must not touch the animal. Check whether any local guidelines are available, if so ensure they are followed. Confirm that there are hand washing facilities available and ensure children wash their hands after handling animals.

- If parents/carers are coming they will need information regarding their role in the outing, the aims and the rules of management of children other than their own and the dos and don'ts of safe group behaviour.

KEY POINT

Regular informal outings to parks and play areas with one baby or a toddler will not require such elaborate arrangements. However, the principles of safety awareness and anticipation of hazards, together with necessary parental agreement will be unchanged.

During the outing

Meticulous planning will limit the chance of anything going wrong. Always allow for children's excitement, so remain calm, and repeat expectations of behaviour and safety rules clearly before departure. Younger children may need some identification of their group, for example a red badge, but not their name or address. Introduce the specific adult who will be in charge of a child or group of children well before you leave. Remind older children of what you want them to gain and achieve.

All children must be kept safe on outings, but within a context of stimulating and encouraging their interests. Outings are an extension of the learning experience so encourage participation, involvement and enthusiasm. On return, ensure older children extend and develop their experience with discussion and associated project and art work.

KEY POINT

Expect the unexpected and be prepared.

Activities

1 Plan and carry out an outing for a group of four-year-olds.
   a) Using a diary format, record your organisation.
   b) Devise information and permission letters for parents.
   c) List the learning outcomes both you and the children should achieve.
   d) Identify special safety features of which you need to be aware for your chosen trip.
   e) How could you extend the learning an outing of this type might provide?
2 Write an evaluation of the plan, its implementation and any changes you would make in future excursions.

QUICK CHECKS

1 Why is knowledge of child development important when planning a safe environment?
2 Why does a baby take objects to her mouth and what safety issues does this 'mouthing' pose?
3 At what developmental stage will a child use the furniture to support her and help her move around a room?
4 When would you say 'no' to a baby and why should you limit the numbers of times you say 'no' to her?
5 Why do you think children with special needs may be particularly vulnerable to accidents?
6 Give three ways you can introduce the idea of safety to a nine-month-old child.
7 How can you use planning and distraction techniques to keep a toddler safe and limit her frustration?
8 What might a toddler do to reach a forbidden object out of immediate range?

9 Why do you consider the need for immediate gratification is potentially hazardous for children and at what age does this lessen?

10 Why may dogs and cats find toddlers frightening and be potentially harmful?

11 At what developmental stage is it realistic for children to have information about keeping safe from strangers?

12 When would you expect a child to be able to listen to instructions whilst involved in an activity?

13 Discuss peer pressure amongst children at Key Stage 1 and consider the implications for safety.

14 Describe five ways of offering safe challenges to a child of seven to satisfy her desire for excitement.

15 At what age do most safety groups think a child might cycle on quiet roads?

16 Why is the Green Cross Code not suitable for children at Key Stage 1?

17 List three reasons why outings with children may be potentially hazardous.

18 Why is it important to have pre-knowledge of a venue for a safe outing?

19 What information do you need from parents/carers before taking a child on an outing?

20 What special developmental factors would you need to take into account when planning outings for toddlers?

4. ACCIDENT PREVENTION

> **This chapter covers:**
> - **Burns, scalds and electric shock**
> - **Falls and cuts**
> - **Sunburn and heatstroke**
> - **Choking, suffocation and drowning**
> - **Poisoning**
> - **Feeding, mealtimes and cooking activities**
> - **Toys and play materials**
> - **Lifting and handling**
> - **Children with special needs**

This chapter discusses a wide range of accident prevention measures. The information can be selected for use in day care and education settings as well as in the home. Remember to cross reference this information with child development in chapter 3 and First Aid practice in chapter 8.

Burns, scalds and electric shock

It is generally acknowledged that burn and scald accidents are linked to poor housing, over-crowding and stress. They are also linked to a child's developmental stage and, as babies become toddlers, curious to explore their environment and discover and experiment, the risk of accidents increases. Children also imitate their carers, so poor or dangerous adult practice will be copied.

Low flammability regulations for nightdresses, the move from open fires to central heating, smoke alarms and improved fireguards have all helped to reduce the number of injuries and deaths from thermal (heat) burns. However, house fires are still a particular danger for all young children – they will have difficulty in escaping from the fire, probably panicking and hiding from the danger.

Chemical burns can be caused by household products such as bleach, oven cleaner and paint stripper – substances which are likely to be in the average home. These burns develop more slowly than thermal burns but can be very serious.

Scalds (injuries caused by hot liquids and steam) mostly affect the face, neck, arms and chest, but can cover the whole body if caused by hot bath water.

Burns and scalds to the mouth and throat may rapidly cause inflammation and swelling of the air passages with a grave risk of suffocation.

The 220 volt domestic electricity supply (in electric sockets, flexes and lighting circuits) can kill or severely burn a child or adult if they come into contact with it, unless the circuits are protected by a Residual Current Device (RCD) which cuts out the supply within a fraction of a second of contact. All day care settings, schools and (preferably) all homes should have the electric circuits protected by RCDs.

PREVENTION OF BURNS

DO

- Use fixed fireguards (British Standard) in the nursery and home. Place a fixed fireguard around a glass fronted fire – the temperature of the glass can reach 250°C causing severe pain and injury if a child touches, or falls against it.
- Install smoke alarms.
- Keep cots away from radiators – a baby can receive a burn to an arm or a leg if a radiator is within reach. Install radiator guards.
- Keep matches and lighters out of children's sight and reach.
- Check upholstered furniture has passed the 'cigarette and match' test.
- Use blinds rather than curtains if the kitchen window is near the cooker.
- Keep a fire blanket in the kitchen and know how to use it.
- Follow fireworks instructions carefully and keep children, well supervised, at a safe distance.
- Carefully supervise celebrations of light, such as Divali and Hanukah, where candles are used.
- Use a coiled flex, or cordless, iron. Never leave an iron switched on and unattended. Unplug and place out of a child's reach to cool down. An unplugged iron remains hot for a considerable time. Wall mounted iron holders are useful.
- Ironing boards can be unstable. It is preferable to iron when the children are not around, or use a kitchen surface or table.
- Keep all household cleaning products and DIY substances locked safely away.
- Check locations of emergency exits when visiting museums, cinemas, theatres etc. with children.

DO NOT

- smoke near children, or leave a burning cigarette in an ashtray anywhere near them
- use portable oil or gas heaters in bathrooms or children's bedrooms
- put clothes on top of fireguards.

PREVENTION OF SCALDS

DO

- Keep teapots, coffee pots, mugs of tea and coffee away from the edge of tables and ledges. Mugs are safer than cups as they have a wider base.

- Keep kettles out of reach – use a coiled flex.
- Fill a kettle with only the amount of water required.
- Keep children away from hot/boiling water and oil. (A chip pan is the most common cause of a kitchen fire. If the pan catches fire turn off the heat, cover the pan with a lid, fire blanket or wet cloth. If you cannot control the fire get out of the kitchen, close the door and call the fire brigade. Preferably, a thermostatically controlled fryer should be used in settings where there are young children).
- Put cold water in the bath first. Test the temperature with your elbow before a child gets in. The water should feel pleasantly warm. A hot water thermostat in the home set to 50°C (129°F) will reduce the risk of scalding. Cover the hot tap with a cloth.

DO NOT

- take hot water into the nursery to heat up feeds
- heat up a baby's bottle in the microwave (see chapter 4, page 91)
- use tablecloths when babies and young children are around to grab the cloth and pull hot food and drink down on themselves. Use table mats if necessary
- pass hot or boiling liquids over a child
- have a hot drink in your hand with a baby or child on your lap
- take hot drinks into the nursery, playroom or classroom or leave them on a surface on to which a child can reach or climb
- leave a young child alone in a kitchen
- add hot water when a child is in the bath
- use showers for young children – the temperature is often difficult to control and bursts of hot water may occur.

KEY POINT

A mug of tea or coffee can remain hot enough to scald a child for up to twenty minutes after being made. A kettle of boiled water is still hot enough to scald one hour after boiling.

Cookers

Cookers can be the source of both burn and scald injuries.

DO

- Use cooker guards or hob guards.
- Keep saucepan handles turned inwards and use back burners whenever possible.
- Switch off electric cookers at wall when not in use.
- Be careful with ceramic hobs – it may be hard to see when the rings are on.
- Secure toddlers in high chairs or in a playpen away from all heat sources.
- Remember that cooker knobs which are out of reach or have to be pushed in to operate are safest.

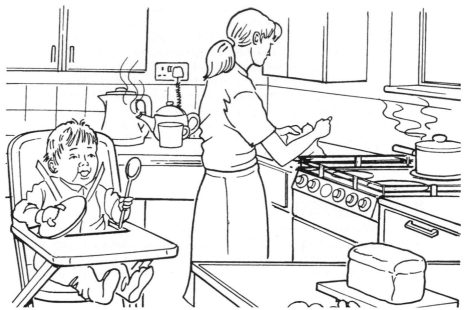

Examples of safe practice to prevent scald injuries – a cooker guard; saucepan on the back burner; kettle, mug and teapot out of reach; toddler secure in his high chair

- allow children to climb anywhere near a cooker
- strain hot foods (such as vegetables or pasta) with a child near your feet.

PREVENTION OF ELECTRIC SHOCK

- Use BEAB approved heating appliances.
- Fit safety covers over electric sockets to prevent children poking an object into them.
- Unplug all electrical appliances when not in use (especially at night).
- Make sure there is always a bulb in lights accessible to children.
- Replace worn out or frayed flexes. A flex so worn that wires are protruding is very dangerous.
- Ensure flexes are correctly connected to plugs and appliances.
- Avoid overloading sockets – a fire could start.
- Find out if electric circuits are protected by an RCD – it is easy for an electrician to fit one in the fuse box.
- Learn to wire up a plug correctly and safely.

Falls and cuts

Falls are the most common accidents in childhood. Once babies are mobile –
wriggling and rolling – they can fall off a changing surface, work surface or a
bed. Toddlers, initially uncoordinated in their movements, run and climb
everywhere in their eagerness to explore the environment. They bump into
things, trip up, fall off a chair, bed or settee but usually end up with nothing
more than a few bruises. However, falling down stairs can result in serious
injury or even death. Falls in gardens where there may be steps, uneven paths,
broken paving stones, footholds for climbing, split-level areas and low walls can
also be serious.

Glass is a major hazard. Ordinary glass can fracture into spear-like shards
inflicting severe pierce injuries or even causing death. Laminated safety glass
will crack, but does not break up when struck or when a child runs into it.
Toughened safety glass can shatter into very small pieces which can inflict
minor, but not usually serious, injuries. Frosted and patterned glass is not
safety glass.

Cut injuries are also caused by sharp knives, scissors, razors, and a range of
gardening implements.

The following reminders identify safe practice to prevent these accidents.

PREVENTION OF FALLS

DO

- Remember to wear appropriate clothes, footwear and jewellery (see chapter
  1, page 5).
- Use a step ladder to reach high windows or objects.
- Keep stairs well lit and clutter free.
- Use stair gates (top and bottom) once a baby is mobile.
- Teach children how to climb up and down steps and stairs safely and to use
  hand rails and banisters.
- Check stair and floor coverings for frayed or worn areas, or turned up cor-
  ners. Ensure that rugs are non-slip and that floors are not highly polished.

Can you identify ten possible hazards?

Reproduced by kind permission of CACHE

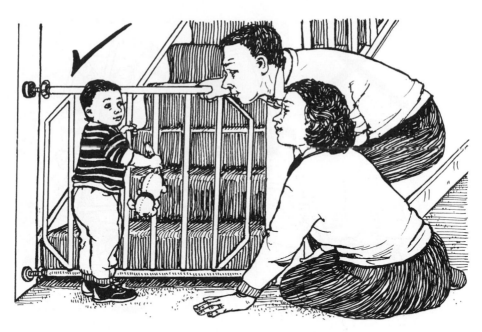

Safe practice – a stair gate in place

- Clean up spills immediately.
- Make sure cots, prams, buggies, high chairs and all harnesses conform to current safety standards. Check regularly for any sign of wear or damage.
- Always use a fixed safety harness in a pram, buggy and high chair.
- Regularly check pram and buggy brakes on a slope.
- Raise cot sides when in use, check safety catches are in working order and nuts and bolt secure.
- Supervise older children lifting a baby out of his cot.
- Check bunk beds (BSEN 747-1) – the gap between the mattress and the rail should not be more than 7.5cm (3in) to prevent a child's head becoming trapped. Children under six years should not sleep in the top bunk.
- Ensure children's clothing is secure and comfortable. Well fitting, securely fastened footwear (especially when outdoors) is essential.
- Teach children to carry items safely and carefully and never to run with anything in their mouths or when carrying glass objects, toys, scissors or other pointed objects.
- Check all climbing equipment is stable, developmentally appropriate, well maintained and properly supervised when in use.
- Make sure there is no crowding on the steps of slides and bars of climbing frames.
- Teach children to wait for the slide to clear before they go down and wait for the swing to stop before they get off.

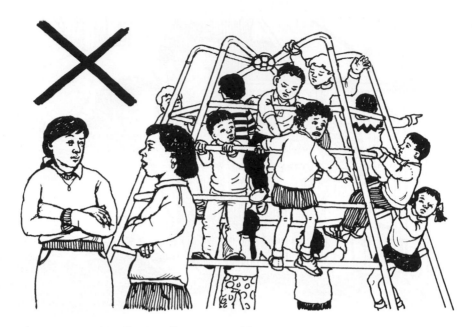

A dangerous and professionally unacceptable situation

- Make steep steps in gardens inaccessible to children.
- Fit child-proof safety catches on windows (especially upstairs) to stop windows opening more than 10cm (4in) (see chapter 5, page 109).
- Help children to take acceptable risks sensibly

(see chapter 5, page 109)

DO NOT

- climb onto a chair or table to reach up high (especially to reach windows), it is dangerous practice which children will copy
- leave a baby where she can roll off a raised edge (bed, table or other surface)
- place a baby in a bouncing cradle on a table top or work surface
- carry more than one baby at a time, or run with a baby (except in a life-threatening emergency)
- place babies in baby walkers nor recommend them to parents (see chapter 3, page 54)
- leave anything a child can climb onto near a window or balcony. Horizontal bars on banisters can be boarded up. Keep balcony doors locked, board up the railings or cover with wire netting.

KEY POINT

If a child wears inappropriate clothing or footwear in the nursery or school, talk to the parents and suggest they bring in alternative items for their child to wear during the day. You can dress him in his 'home' clothes or shoes before he leaves the setting.

PREVENTION OF CUTS

DO

- Make sure glass in doors and windows where children can bump into them is laminated or toughened to 76cm (2ft 6in) above floor level, unless fire regulations require the use of wired glass or copper light glazing in doors. Glass in book-cases and glass topped tables may need to be replaced with safety glass or covered with safety film. Highlight low level windows and patio doors with coloured strips to prevent children running into them.
- Keep razors, scissors, knives, woodwork tools and other sharp objects well out of a young child's sight and reach. Carefully supervise children using sharp knives during cooking activities, scissors during cutting activities and various tools during woodwork activities. Only adults should use a staple gun.
- Check outdoor areas for broken glass, jagged drinks cans, rusty nails, and so on before allowing children out to play.
- Wrap broken glass carefully in newspaper before placing it in the dustbin.

DO NOT

- allow children to run when carrying sharp or glass objects.

Activity

Observe a group of no more than four young children aged eighteen months to two and a half years playing over a period of 20 minutes. Make notes of how many times each child engages in a climbing activity, for example up or down steps or stairs, into a chair, on to a carer's lap, or into or out of a box. Write up your findings in graph or chart form.

Sunburn and heatstroke

Children's skin is delicate and sensitive. It will easily and quickly burn if exposed to direct sunlight on a hot day (especially if it is windy as well).

Heatstroke occurs as a result of excessive heat. A child with heatstroke may or may not have sunburn.

SUNBURN

Sunburn causes soreness and reddening of the skin (not immediately apparent) and may be followed by blistering and bleeding. Severe sunburn leaves a child feeling unwell, dehydrated and in pain. Research shows that early exposure to hot sun, particularly when reflected off sea and sand, can cause skin cancer in later life. Sunscreen products will afford protection only if they are adequately applied to the skin.

Asian, African and children of mixed race, as well as white children all need protection from the sun.

HEATSTROKE

Too much sun can be very serious in babies and young children as they are unable to regulate their body temperature. A child with heatstroke will typically:

- look flushed and feel very hot
- have a raised temperature and rapid pulse
- be dehydrated
- appear confused with uncoordinated movements.

He may also develop a pin-point, red heat rash.

In serious cases of heatstroke a child can fall into a coma and die. Any baby or child developing signs of heatstroke must be seen by a doctor. In the meantime, cool him slowly by tepid sponging. Apply calamine lotion to the rash if it is itchy. A baby who is over-dressed or wrapped up too tightly and warmly may also develop heatstroke.

To prevent sunburn and heatstroke and to keep young children comfortable on hot days follow the good practice set out below.

CARE OF CHILDREN IN THE SUN

DO

- Keep babies under six months in the shade at all times.
- Place a baby's pram in the shade, watch as the sun moves round and change the pram position accordingly. Pram canopies afford more protection than parasols.
- Dress babies and older children in cool, closely woven clothing (special sun protection clothing is available) and wide brimmed hats, or French Legion style ones with a visor and protection for ears and neck. The back of the neck, shoulders, tops of arms and thighs must be covered. Make sure children are covered up when playing in the sea or paddling pool on a hot day. A baby's bottom can readily burn, so if you remove a nappy, replace it with a pair of cotton pants.
- Use a hypoallergenic water resistant sunblock cream of at least SPF (Sun Protection Factor) 25, from a range especially for children (Sun E45 SPF 25 and 50). Apply generously before children go outside, whether children are wearing protective clothes or not. Remember the neck and tops of the ears. Re-apply sunblock every 2 to 3 hours, after paddling or swimming and towelling a child dry. An 'aftersun' product can be applied when they return indoors. Check the date on sunblock products – an out-of-date cream can result in burning. The Child Accident Prevention Trust advises parents and carers to check with the health visitor about which sunblock to use.
- Re-apply sunblock after paddling or swimming.

- Encourage children to drink plenty water on a hot day to prevent dehydration. Offer babies cooled, boiled water.
- Schedule indoor routines and activities for when the sun is at its hottest (11 am–3 pm). Open the windows, use a fan (placed in a very safe place) to provide a cooling draught.
- Make the most of naturally shaded areas when children are playing outside. Create temporary shaded areas with parasols, tents or covered dens.

Carers may assume, wrongly, that an application of sunblock is sufficient protection for children. Keeping children in the shade, dressing them in cool, protective clothing and avoiding the midday sun are essential measures. The well-known slogan: 'Slip, Slop, Slap' – slip on a shirt, slop on some sun cream and slap on a hat – is a useful reminder of safe practice in the sun.

Sunglasses for children should conform to BS2724 which means they have the required UV (ultraviolet) filters.

KEY POINTS

- Nursery and school staff should follow their local authority guidelines about applying sunscreen products to children.
- If a child is allergic to sunscreen products, the parents should talk to the family doctor or health visitor.

Activity
Design a frieze for your nursery to raise awareness of the dangers of the sun, and the steps carers can take to protect children in hot, sunny weather.

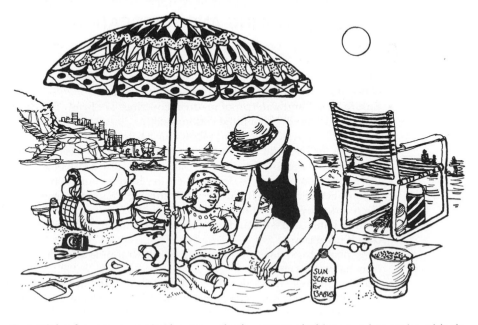

Essential safety measures in the sun – shade, cotton clothing, sun hat and sunblock

Choking, suffocation and drowning

By around the age of four to six months, everything a baby can reach and grasp is taken to his mouth. A baby or young child may choke on ribbons and ties on clothing, toy parts, beads and bits of jewellery, marbles, peanuts, hard pieces of food and, particularly in babies, regurgitated food. Some of these objects may be inhaled causing lung infection or even death. Crumbly foods may increase the risk of choking in children with cerebral palsy.

Smooth objects which are swallowed often pass through the digestive tract without too much difficulty, although button batteries, used in many watches and calculators, contain mercury which can be poisonous if absorbed into the body. Sharp objects such as brooches or badges with open pins can cause internal injury.

Suffocation can be caused by pillows, baby nests, duvets and uncovered plastic mattresses, plastic bags and wrappings and pets overlaying a baby. A baby or young child may also suffocate if he becomes overheated in a cot, bed, pram or car.

Most ball point pen tops, which can easily be swallowed, and plastic shopping bags now have ventilation holes.

Babies and young children can drown very quickly in just 3cm (1¼in) of water. All water sources, including pools or ponds, buckets and bowls of water left unattended, puddles and bird baths are potentially dangerous.

The following lists identify safe practice to prevent these accidents.

PREVENTION OF CHOKING AND SUFFOCATION

DO

- Check cot mattresses meet BS1877 (see chapter 2, page 46). Large gaps between mattress and cot could trap a baby's head.
- Ensure plastic and waterproof mattress coverings are firmly fitted, securely fixed and covered with a fitted cotton sheet.
- Avoid cot bumpers, duvets and pillows for a baby under one year. A baby would be unable to lift his head or wriggle free if his face became 'buried' in, or pressed against, the soft material. There is also a risk of overheating.
- Place a baby on his back to sleep and ensure he does not get trapped under the covers (see Sudden Infant Death Syndrome, chapter 5, page 124).
- Keep cots away from windows and heaters. Make sure a baby cannot reach a window blind cord – it could get wrapped around his neck. Shorten the cord if necessary.
- Keep plastic bags, flimsy dry-cleaning plastic wrapping and cling film away from babies and children.
- Use cat and insect nets when babies sleep outside. Bee and wasp stings around the mouth can cause swelling and inflammation of the air passages. A cat can smother a baby.
- Keep pets and domestic animals out of children's bedrooms.

- Check all toys for safety and condition (especially if second-hand). Look for the Lion Mark and BSEN number.
- Keep mobiles away from a baby's face.
- Avoid soft toys made with inferior fur which can be pulled or bitten off causing choking. Furry toys are not suitable for children under one year.

DO NOT

- hang blankets around cot sides.
- dress a baby in fussy clothes. Ties and ribbons should be no longer than 20cm (8in)
- attach dummies to a baby's clothes with a string longer than 20cm (8in)
- put babies outside to sleep in very cold, foggy or wet weather
- 'prop feed' a baby or leave an older baby alone with finger foods, especially hard foods such as pieces of apple, carrot or cheese
- give children hard boiled sweets
- give peanuts to children under five years. Check for nut (especially peanut) allergy.

KEY POINTS

- All babies sleeping outside in a day care setting should be checked every ten minutes to make sure they are well and warm, but not overheated. Make sure a written, signed record is made of every check.
- Check that you understand the First Aid procedures for choking in both a baby and child (see chapter 8, page 207).

WATER SAFETY AND PREVENTION OF DROWNING

DO

- Place locks on the outside of bathroom doors high up out of children's reach.
- Support and securely hold onto babies in the bath, especially the older babies who wriggle, twist and try to stand. Use a rubber safety mat.
- Stay with children under four years all the time they are in the bath.
- Drain or fill in garden ponds until young children are able to understand the dangers, or cover with rigid mesh which is securely anchored, fenced off to a height of 1.5m (5ft) and checked frequently for signs of damage.
- Closely supervise children near a garden pond, even if it mesh-covered.
- Keep water butts (or other rain water containers) tightly covered and fenced off.
- Empty buckets and other water containers immediately after use.
- Teach children the dangers of walking too near the edges of any water source.
- Stay with children using a paddling pool. Immediately after use, drain it well and turn it upside down. Drain any rain water which may accumulate on top of it.

- Securely cover and fence off an outdoor swimming pool (it can be dangerous both empty and full). Check the fence regularly. Keep the gate in the fence locked. Keep the door to an indoor pool locked.
- Maintain a carer:child ratio of 1:1 for under fives, and 1:2 for children aged five to eight years in a swimming pool or at the seaside. Stay with the children at all times. Make sure those who cannot swim wear buoyancy aids and remain within their safe standing depth.
- Check in a swimming pool that:
  - lifeguards are on duty
  - bather operated alarms are installed and in working order
  - all 'danger' signs are clearly written and visible.
- Carefully supervise children on a water slide – accidents happen when the slides are very busy and there is crowding, particularly at 'splash down'.
- Teach children to swim, float, tread water and feel confident in water.
- Make sure children wear life jackets during any water sports.
- Check with public health authorities for clean, safe beaches and sea.

DO NOT

- leave babies and young children under four years alone in the bath, even for a few seconds
- let children play unattended in the bathroom
- allow children to walk on pond, river or canal ice – it is rarely thick enough in the UK to support weight and the water will be extremely cold and may be very deep
- allow children to swim in rivers and canals
- allow children near the sea unattended
- leave children playing alone in rock pools.

Activity
You are making a pre-visit to the local swimming pool to discuss booking a session for a group of children aged two to three years. Describe the safety measures you would expect to find in place to prevent accidents both in the water and in the changing area.

Poisoning

The risk of a poisoning accident is greatest at times of illness, stress and disruption in the home. Common substances that children take are medicines, tablets and household cleaners. To young children, prescribed and 'over the counter' (OTC) medicines look like something interesting to drink, and pills or tablets resemble small sweets. Parents, relatives, visitors to the home and others may inadvertently leave medication in handbags, in the kitchen or bathroom, or on bedside tables. Iron tablets, frequently prescribed for anaemia and for women during pregnancy, can, if ingested by a child cause internal bleeding and intestinal and kidney damage. Chewing cigarette ends can cause vomiting and 'nicotine rushes' in a child. Mouthwashes are often brightly coloured and appear attractive. They look harmless and are not required to have child resistant caps, but they can contain high levels of alcohol.

Under eighteen months, children lack refined good or bad taste discrimination, and may swallow substances an older child or adult would spit out. Older children may encourage or 'dare' others into tasting something poisonous.

Dangerous household products must never be within reach of young children. They include: bleach, disinfectants, detergents, lavatory cleaner, caustic soda, turpentine, weed killer, paraffin, methylated spirit, battery acid, slug pellets, rat poison, insecticides, DIY substances, perfumes, nail varnish remover, marker pens and alcohol.

KEY POINT

Whenever possible, make sure medicines, tablets, pills and household products are in containers with child resistant caps. These caps have markedly reduced the incidence of poisoning in children since they were introduced in the mid-1970s.

PREVENTION OF POISONING

The following reminders identify good practice to prevent poisoning accidents.

Plants, shrubs, berries, fungi

DO

- Warn children not to eat plants, leaves, mushrooms, toadstools or berries. Laburnum leaves and seeds, holly berries, lupin seeds and laurel leaves are very poisonous. Some house plants can be dangerous if eaten.

KEY POINT

Although rhubarb, tomato and potato leaves are poisonous, they can be grown in cages where children cannot reach them.

Medicines, pills and tablets

DO

- Keep pills, tablets and medicines in child resistant containers, out of sight and reach in a locked cupboard. Remind visitors to keep their medication out of children's reach.
- Keep mouth washes locked away, they contain alcohol.
- Return all unused medicines and pills to the chemist or flush them down the lavatory.

- transfer pills from one container to another.

Alcohol

DO

- Treat alcohol as a poison and keep it locked away.
- Keep an alcoholic drink out of a child's reach.

Household products

DO

- Keep all household products and DIY substances in their original containers in locked cupboards out of children's reach.
- Keep garden sheds and garages locked.

DO NOT

- mix bleach with lavatory cleaner (see chapter 2, page 36)
- put dangerous substances such as weed killer in a familiar container (e.g. a lemonade bottle) which a child could presume was all right to drink.

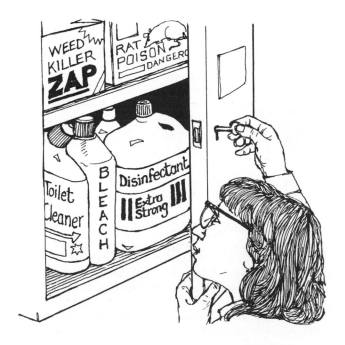

Keep dangerous substances in a locked cupboard

Materials for children's activities

> ■ Make sure crayons, paints, glues and colourings used in a wide range of activities are non-toxic.
> ■ Discourage children from putting paint brushes, crayons, dough and Plasticine etc. in their mouths.

KEY POINTS

- ■ Lead paint on old toys and nursery equipment, or sometimes on new, cheap, imported toys sold in street markets and car boot sales, can be ingested if young children suck, bite and chew toys.
- ■ Natural remedies may be toxic to a child. Keep them locked up out of reach, just as you would prescribed medicines.

Carbon monoxide

Carbon monoxide poisoning can occur if gas heating appliances (gas fires, central heating units, gas water heaters, living-flame fires) are used in a poorly ventilated room or the flue is obstructed. Regular checks should be made on equipment and repair work carried out by a CORGI registered fitter. By law there must be an annual service for gas appliances in nursery or school premises.

Feeding, mealtimes and cooking activities

FEEDING

Safe practice when preparing feeds and feeding babies includes high standards of hygiene to prevent infection and measures to prevent choking or scalding accidents.

SAFE AND HYGIENIC PRACTICE WHEN PREPARING FEEDS AND FEEDING BABIES

> ■ Store dried milks in a cool, dry place and check sell-by date before use.
> ■ Prepare feeds away from young children, using formula consistent with the parent's wishes and any medical advice. Nurseries should have a separate milk kitchen close to the baby and toddler room.
> ■ Thoroughly clean the feed preparation area – floor, work surfaces, sinks, taps and kettle.
> ■ Wash all feeding equipment in hot, soapy water and sterilise using a chemical agent (see chapter 2, page 34), steam steriliser or boiling method.
> ■ Wash hands and scrub nails thoroughly with soap and hot water before making up feeds.

ACCIDENT PREVENTION **91**

- Store made-up feeds in a fridge (up to 24 hours) until needed. Fridge temperature should be 3–5°C (37–41°F).
- Check the temperature of the feed on the inside of your wrist before offering it to the baby.
- Check the milk flow, it should be several drops per second – too fast a flow can cause choking.
- Supervise siblings and adults unused to caring for babies when they are feeding a young baby.
- Remove the baby's bib after a feed to prevent it covering his face.
- Throw away any unused feed.

DO NOT

- take hot water into the nursery to warm up feeds
- warm up feeds in a microwave – unexpected 'hot spots' can occur causing a scald injury to the baby's mouth
- 'prop feed' a baby (a baby is left alone with a bottle propped up in his mouth).

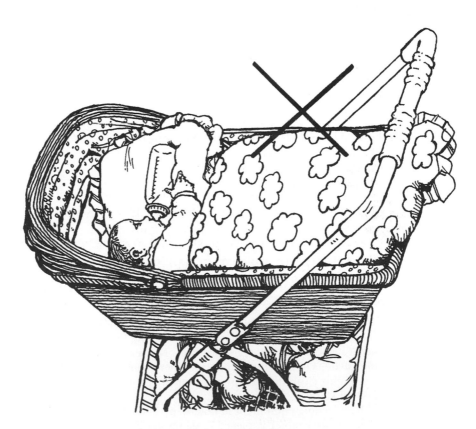

Never leave a baby alone with a feeding bottle propped up in her mouth ('prop' feeding)

KEY POINTS

■ Milk is an ideal medium in which harmful bacteria can breed. Continue to sterilise all feeding equipment (bottles, teats, knives, spoons, jugs) until the baby is one year old.

■ Plates, bowls and drinking cups should be sterilised until the baby is about nine months old, after which they can be kept socially clean (washed up in hot soapy water, rinsed well and left to drain and dry) or washed in the dishwasher.

MEALTIMES

Mealtimes are busy periods whether in a nursery, at school or at home and the potential for accidents is great especially among the younger age groups.

SAFE AND HYGIENIC PRACTICE AT MEALTIMES

DO

- Use high chair harnesses.
- Wipe down high chairs after each use with hot, soapy water and an antiseptic solution. Scrub them thoroughly every week (more often if necessary) and allow them to dry in the fresh air and sunlight whenever possible.
- Keep the eating area (floor, tables and chairs) clean.
- Wipe up spills of food, drink and grease immediately.
- Cut food up into manageable pieces for young children.
- Provide cutlery which a child can easily use.
- Check fish and chicken for bones.
- Check fruit for pips and stones.
- Offer drinks of water in plastic cups or mugs (pieces can be bitten out of glass tumblers).
- Check with parents before offering children peanut butter sandwiches or food containing nuts (but do not give to children under five years).
- Be aware of any food allergies children may have (the foods and the reactions they cause).
- Find out from parents any particular food requirements for children with special needs and the type of bowls and cutlery they can safely manage.
- Store children's packed lunches in the fridge if possible, especially in hot weather. Advise parents about foods which can be safely stored at room temperature.

DO NOT

- leave a baby alone with finger foods
- blow on a baby's food or test the temperature with your finger – always use a separate sterile spoon
- pass food or drink over a child's head – approach from the side
- allow children to walk around whilst eating or drinking
- give whole or broken nuts to children under five years

- give children hard sweets or toffees
- use tablecloths
- leave plastic bread bags or sharp knives on the table where children can get at them.

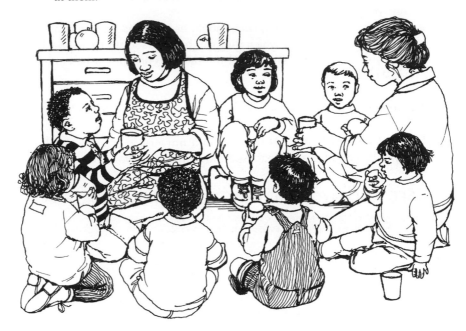

Safe practice – children sitting down to eat and drink and carers approaching from the side when offering children food and drink

KEY POINTS

- Hand washing is essential for carers, babies who are mobile, and children before feeding and mealtimes.
- Children with cerebral palsy often have a poor cough reflex. Avoid offering them crumbly foods such as biscuits or toast which may cause choking.

COOKING ACTIVITIES

Day nurseries, nursery classes and schools are in a position to offer children a variety of cooking experiences in a safe and supervised setting.

Organisation and management
Not more than 4 children under five years, or 6 children between five and seven years, should take part in a cooking activity with one adult. Make sure the children not involved in cooking are engaged in a supervised different activity, so that they are not a safety hazard through boredom or getting in the way. Let them know they will have the chance to cook next time.

There is greater risk of an accident if children become bored or frustrated, so the concentration ability and skill level of the group must be considered. Adaptations to the cooking area and additional help may be needed for children with special needs.

SAFE AND HYGIENIC PRACTICE DURING COOKING ACTIVITIES

The following lists set out safe and hygienic practice during cooking activities.

Preparation of the children

DO

- Ensure children wash their hands thoroughly before and after the activity.
- Check that finger nails are short, no rings are worn, hair is tied back and children's clean aprons put on.
- Explain the safety rules clearly and fully.
- Make sure there are sufficient bowls, spoons and aprons so the children are not bored and restless waiting for a turn.
- Encourage everyone to be involved in clearing away and washing up safely.

The activity

DO

- Make sure the cooking area is clean and uncluttered.
- Maintain supervision and a high staff:child ratio.
- Teach children to use equipment safely e.g. beaters and peelers, and how to cut with a sharp knife.
- Be a role model for safe and hygienic procedures and teach them to the children as part of the cooking activity.
- Keep the First Aid box nearby in case of an accident.

DO NOT

- prepare and cook food to which any child in the group is allergic, or, for any other reason, cannot eat
- allow young children near the heat source. Using oven gloves, and with supervision, older children may place their cooking inside the oven
- let children light a gas oven with matches
- use hot fat or frying methods of cooking with young children
- allow children to pour boiling water
- allow children to taste food without your permission, nor eat food that has fallen onto the floor.

Toys and play materials

Parents, teachers, nursery workers and other carers must make sure that toys provided for children are safe. Toys which are badly made or used inappropriately can be dangerous and cause accidents.

Toys must be strong and stable, clean and hygienic, free from dyes which rub off and free from lead in paint coatings. They must not present a fire risk. There must be no sharp edges or points and any detachable parts must be too big to swallow. Packaging, especially plastic bags which could cause suffocation, must be disposed of safely. Materials such as paints, crayons, felt pens, colourings, dough and Plasticine, glues and art and craft products must all be non-toxic. It is important to follow the instructions provided with a toy or other materials.

Toys marked BSEN71–BS5665 have met the highest British and European Union Safety requirements for toys. Care should be taken when buying toys at doubtful outlets as they may not bear authorised markings.

Whilst the age range for which the manufacturer considers a toy suitable and safe is shown on the packaging, a child's developmental stage must also be considered.

Toys are dropped in food, put in potties or down the lavatory and thrown out of prams and pushchairs. They get dirty and harbour germs. They are chewed and explored in the mouth (especially in the first eighteen months). Make sure toys are kept clean and hygienic, especially those used by babies.

Phthalates

Chemicals called phthalates (pronounced 'thalates') soften the hard substance polyvinyl chloride (PVC) so that it moulds easily. Sucking and chewing on PVC toys, such as teething rings and rattles, causes the chemicals to leach out and be swallowed by the child. Current concerns link the amounts of phthalates leaching out to health problems such as liver and kidney disease and testicular cancer. A European Union emergency ban is now in place on PVC teething toys. Further legislation for a permanent ban is proposed but this will take time for the European Parliament to enact. Whilst many toys are now made from alternative plastics always find out from the retailer or supplier if they contain phthalates and look for non-PVC products.

TOY SAFETY AND HYGIENE

The following lists set out safety and hygiene considerations for toys and play materials.

Safety

DO

- Make sure toys are safe and developmentally appropriate. Look for the sign indicating a toy is unsafe for children 0–3 years.
- Check that young children cannot get at small removable parts.

- Supervise children when they are playing with beads, buttons and small Lego pieces – they may put them in ears, up noses or swallow them.
- Store toys safely at a low level, never on high shelves.
- Purpose-built storage boxes must have lids which will not trap fingers or close completely, so trapping a child who might be hiding inside.
- Make sure toys are not left lying on the stairs.
- Check toys daily for damage – some may be mended successfully and safely, otherwise throw them away. Remove a broken toy as soon as it is discovered.
- Encourage children to identify any toys which are broken.
- Check wooden toys, bricks and blocks for splinters.
- Check soft and furry toys for BSEN71–BS5665 number – it would indicate fur and fillings are safe. Make sure eyes are firmly fixed and secure.
- Teach children to play with toys in the way that is recommended, not to be destructive or aggressive with them.
- Support children in helping to tidy toys away. This encourages care and respect for them, and helps to prevent accidents.

Toys for babies

DO

- Check there are no small parts which can become loose and swallowed or inhaled.
- Check toys are not so hard as to hurt if dropped on fingers or toes.
- Carefully supervise a baby playing with paper – he may chew off and choke on small pieces.

DO NOT

- give furry toys to babies under one year
- attach toys on a string round a baby's neck or give babies toys with long narrow parts which could reach the back of a baby's mouth.

Hygiene

DO

- Wash and scrub toys weekly in hot, soapy water and antiseptic, rinse and dry well. Soft toys, material books and bricks can be washed by hand or machine washed. When possible allow them to dry in the fresh air and sunlight.
- Wash and sterilise teething rings and rattles every day.
- Sterilise dummies after each use. Babies must have their own dummies kept in individual containers until required.

LOCAL AUTHORITY MONITORING

Trading Standards Officers:
- regularly test sample toys for flammability, adequacy of instructions and warnings, fillings in soft toys
- investigate complaints about toys
- have powers to stop the sale of dangerous toys.

Activity

Research the safety information and signs on a variety of toys in the following ways.

a) List toys and games typically used in a nursery setting, for example, soft toys, Duplo, Lego, wooden and plastic bricks, musical boxes, posting boxes, sorting and matching games, puzzles etc.

b) Visit local toy retail outlets and identify the safety information and signs on your listed toys and games. Look for the BSEN71–BS5665 number, the Lion Mark and 'Age Warning' symbol.

c) Place the appropriate safety indicator against each toy.

d) Visit a toy stall in your local street market. Identify toys similar to the ones on your list. Do they all carry one of the recognised safety marks?

e) Look at rattles and teething rings. Do any of them say 'PVC free'?

PLAY MATERIALS – SAFETY AND HYGIENE

Water, painting, drawing and messy activities

DO

- Protect children's clothing, the floor and table tops. Wipe up spills as soon as they occur.
- Check for allergies if you are adding colouring to water or other messy materials, or perfumes or soaps to water.
- Start a water play session with clean, warm water in the tray. Change it or top it up as necessary. Equipment and toys used during play must be in good condition and washed after every session.
- Remove pen tops before children draw or colour in.

DO NOT

- allow children to drink the water or suck their fingers, put paint brushes in their mouths, or eat dough, cornflour or other similar materials
- allow children to put pencils in their mouths.

Sand

DO

- Keep sand clean. Sieve and wash spilt sand to remove dirt and grit, or throw it away.
- Keep an outdoor sand pit securely covered when not in use to prevent contamination from animal fouling and other debris.

- allow children to throw or eat sand (it can cause eye irritation and choking).

KEY POINTS

- Sand is difficult to remove from tight, curly hair and can lead to scalp irritation and infection. A child may need to wear a hat or head scarf during sand play to avoid these risks.
- Make sure children wash their hands thoroughly after playing with sand and messy materials.

Woodwork, construction and craft activities

- Supervise children closely when they are using woodwork tools, scissors or needles. Only older children should have access to woodwork tools.
- Remember, children should be in small, well supervised groups when playing with small items such as beads and buttons.

- leave any tools or small items lying around, store them carefully after use
- allow children to throw or play roughly with large construction blocks.

KEY POINT

Children with eczema and other skin conditions may need to wear gloves when using art and craft paints and glues, and malleable or messy materials.

Dressing-up clothes

- Wash dressing-up clothes weekly or monthly, depending on their use. Always wash them if there is an outbreak of infection such as diarrhoea and vomiting, scabies or impetigo.

Lifting and handling

Employers have a responsibility to reduce, as far as possible, the risk of injury to their employees and provide advice and training in correct techniques when lifting duties are integral to the workplace activities. The local authority environmental health department, St John Ambulance and physiotherapists can offer appropriate advice and suggest suitable training organisations.

Back injuries as a result of lifting incorrectly are common and once damage is done to the spine and its supporting structures (muscles and ligaments) there is always a risk of further injury in the weakened area. There are several things you can do to help keep your back in good condition

■ Maintain your ideal weight and adopt good posture – avoid slouching and hunching your shoulders.
■ Take regular exercise to keep your muscles toned.
■ Sleep on a firm, well sprung mattress and firm base. Try to use only one pillow – too many will put a twist on the neck.
■ Avoid curling up in soft, easy chairs. More upright chairs provide support for the lower back and prevent backache.
■ Avoid carrying babies, bags or parcels on one hip – it may cause a sideways tilt to your spine.
■ Wear comfortable and supportive footwear. High heels push the body's centre of gravity forward, they also contribute to accidents.

Child care duties will include lifting children, nursery and school furniture, play equipment and so on. Think carefully about tasks which involve stooping, reaching upwards, twisting, lifting, lowering, carrying for long distances, or excessive pushing or pulling. Light lifting tasks should present little difficulty. For heavier lifting tasks follow the steps below.

LIFTING TECHNIQUE

a) Assess what needs to be lifted (the load). Is it heavy – can you make it lighter or reduce the weight or size? Is it bulky – can you make it smaller? Is it difficult to grasp – can you attach handles? Can you share the lifting with others?
b) Stand close to the load with feet apart for good balance.
c) Bend your knees, keep your back straight and straddle the load.
d) Grip the load securely (accidents frequently occur when the load slips from hands).
e) Lift slowly, avoiding jerky movements. Straighten your knees and stand.

REMEMBER

The nearer to your body you carry the load the less strain you place on your back. Aim to reduce the risk of injury by:
■ using your body more efficiently
■ team handling
■ re-planning the lifting task.

KEY POINTS

■ If two or more people are lifting together, make sure they are of similar height and decide who will give the commands. If a load is too heavy and no one is available to help you, do not lift it – wait for help.
■ Carers who are unwell or pregnant should not lift heavy loads.

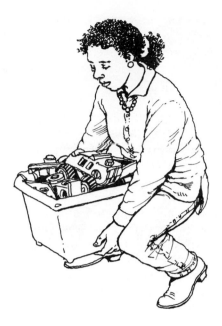

Always remember to lift correctly

LIFTING AND HANDLING BABIES AND YOUNG CHILDREN

The bones of babies and young children are easily damaged. The process of calcification (laying down of calcium and hardening) takes place over many years. A baby's head is large and heavy in relation to the rest of his body and must be well supported until his neck muscles are strong enough to maintain support. To prevent the risk of harm or accident when lifting and handling babies and young children follow these guidelines.

- Lift babies and young children gently, carefully and with respect. Jerky or rough handling is frightening and dangerous. Always support a young baby's head.
- Carry a baby close to your body – this makes him feel secure and lessens the strain on your back. You can carry an older baby with your arm around his tummy and his back against your body.
- Never pick up a baby or child, nor swing him round, by his wrists, arms or clothing, it can cause dislocated wrists, elbows and shoulders. Throwing babies in the air as a 'fun' game is also very dangerous.
- When lifting a child, stand as close as possible to him, look at him and tell him what you are going to do. Keep your back straight and hold him firmly and symmetrically around the trunk as you lift.
- Make sure there is no obstruction to impede the lift such as loose clothing, a harness, or dangling jewellery to catch on furniture or bedding
- Carry only one baby at a time, unless there is a life-threatening emergency such as fire.

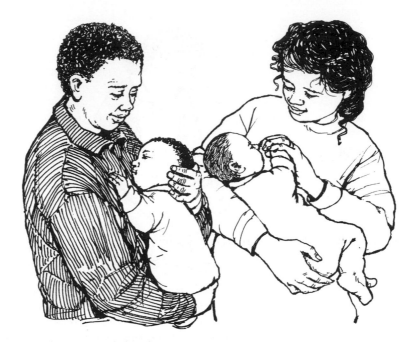

Hold a young baby close to your body, supporting his head at all times

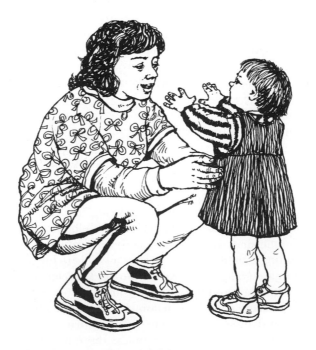

Lift children gently and safely

- Two carers may be needed to lift a child with special needs. Explain to the child what you are doing. Remember to lift as outlined on pages 101–102 – knees bent, back straight, holding the child close to your body.

Always be a role model for correct lifting. Teach children how to lift and carry to protect their backs. Whilst school children should be encouraged to carry their bags on their backs, so distributing the weight evenly, rather than over one shoulder or balanced on one hip, the bags must not be overly heavy.

KEY POINT

Find out from parents if there is a particular way their baby or child prefers to be lifted or handled.

Children with special needs

You may care for children with special needs in your setting. As for all children, safety must be a priority. Liaison between carers and parents is essential – parents know their children best and are experts on their abilities and needs. Planning advice, special alterations and particular resources (including extra staff) may occasionally be necessary, but most early years settings will need only minor adjustments to buildings and only a few children will need special provisions. The emphasis must be on offering safe, good and varied play and education experiences based on individual need and ability. Staff trained in

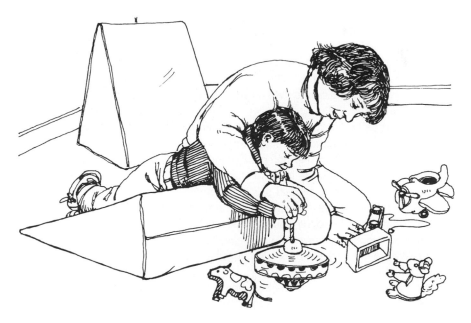

A child with special needs plays with his key worker

inclusive practice are better able to understand and support children with special needs. The registered charity, the Handicapped Adventure Playground Association (HAPA) provides a national training and information service promoting the development of inclusive play and the Disability Resource Team can provide disability equality training. The addresses of both these organisations are on pages 221 and 222.

KEY POINT

An identification bracelet is usually worn by children with diabetes, epilepsy or haemophilia. This is particularly helpful for accident prevention purposes, or if a child becomes unwell in an unexpected situation or new staff are involved in their care.

QUICK CHECKS

1 What four factors have contributed to the reduction of childhood deaths from burns?
2 What precautions would you take to prevent a burn or scald injury when bathing a) a baby b) a young child?
3 For how long can the following remain hot enough to scald, a) a mug of tea or coffee b) a kettle of boiled water?
4 Give three examples of good practice to protect a baby from falling.
5 How can areas of ordinary glass in windows and doors in a setting be made safer for the children?
6 Which areas of a child's skin are particularly vulnerable to sunburn and must always be covered to protect from the sun?
7 Why are cot bumpers, duvets and pillows not recommended for babies under one year?
8 Why is it important to use cat nets on prams when babies are sleeping outside?
9 What is the danger to a child of swallowing a small button battery?
10 What safety precautions would you take to protect a child from drowning at the seaside?
11 What particular safety precautions should be taken with a) a garden pond b) a water butt c) an outdoor swimming pool?
12 Why are mouthwashes potentially dangerous for young children?
13 What particular safety invention has reduced the number of children attending hospital having swallowed pills or tablets?
14 Give three examples of safe practice at mealtimes to prevent a child from choking.
15 What particular foods would you avoid offering a child with cerebral palsy?
16 How would you prevent a scald injury to a baby's mouth from his milk feed?
17 Why might rattles and teething rings be potentially dangerous for babies and young children?
18 When MUST you wash dressing-up clothes?
19 What is the danger of lifting up babies and children by their arms or wrists?
20 For which disorders do children usually wear identification bracelets?

5 SAFE ENVIRONMENTS

> **This chapter covers:**
> - **Nursery and school**
> - **The home**
> - **Holidays**
> - **Cars and minibuses**
> - **Seat belts and child restraint systems**
> - **Community playgrounds**

Children need safe places, indoors and outdoors, in which to live, learn and play, so making their environment as safe as possible is your first priority.

Nursery and school

The nursery and school environment must be welcoming, well ventilated, adequately lit (with as much natural light as possible), and sufficiently spacious for physical exercise and play, and a wide range of focused activities and experiences. Stuffy, cramped, crowded conditions, lead to tiredness, irritability and frustration, all of which present a greater risk of accidents.

SECURING THE PREMISES

The 1996 Government Report, *Improving Security in Schools*, stressed the need for an integrated approach to child safety provision which combines effective vigilance and alertness by management and staff, with a system of physical controls.

Security measures and systems
Whatever systems are used to keep the children safely inside the premises, and intruders, vandals and dogs out, there must be a balance between protecting the children and allowing them freedom and independence. Security systems include the following measures.
- Perimeter fences and walls must be high enough to prohibit children climbing them and have secure gates and entrance and exit doors. No child should be able to wander away from the setting. Emergency escape routes must be maintained, especially where the entrance and exit is limited to one door.
- Safe arrangements must be in place for children's arrival and departure times with a specific routine for handing over a child to someone other than the named person.
- Intruder alarms may be advisable in some areas.

- Electronic systems, being used increasingly in care and education settings, include:
  - closed circuit television (CCTV) cameras, with 24 hour surveillance and recording
  - video entry phones which allow visitors to be seen on screen before they are allowed entry
  - intercoms
  - palm and finger print recognition procedures on entry
  - mobile phones for staff to use when outside the premises with children.

KEY POINT

No child must be able (or allowed) to leave the premises without supervision.

INDOORS AND OUTDOORS

In the interests of health and safety particular attention must be given to:
- carer:child ratio
- alert, responsible supervision and assessment of risks
- emergency escape routes, fire prevention and fire practices
- inclusive access design – the physical, learning and play environments must be accessible to all the children, including children with special needs
- easy access from indoors to the outside play areas and street (for example, keeping paths clear, especially in ice and snow conditions)
- appropriate lighting, heating and ventilation
- safety and maintenance checks of large and small equipment
- safety rules for the children – teaching safe behaviour, how to carry materials and equipment correctly, no running at particular times, and so on
- personal hygiene facilities for babies and children
- cooking facilities and meal time arrangements
- provision for children's rest and sleep
- staff welfare – staff rest room, lavatory and hand washing facilities
- professional practice of 'clearing up as you go'.

Make sure toys and equipment you select for children are:
- manufactured to current safety standards
- appropriate for age, abilities and strength
- stimulating, confidence building and inviting exploration and learning (remember, frustration and boredom lead to accidents)
- a mixture of natural and artificial materials
- durable
- inclusive
- value for money.

REMEMBER

Always read the manufacturer's information and instructions on the packaging of toys and equipment.

INDOORS

Think about your indoor setting.

- Is the entrance welcoming to all – children, staff, parents and visitors?
- Is the setting visually attractive?
- Are the children's rooms – play and classrooms – inviting and interesting, well lit and well laid out?
- Is there child-sized furniture, soft seating and other pieces of furniture which might be used as partitions?
- Is there space available for floor play, sleeping and eating? Separate rooms are ideal for these functions, but in reality they often take place in the same room.
- Are the lavatory and hand washing facilities close to the play and classrooms?

Accidents may occur because of crowding, pushing and general excitement when children are moving from one area to another. Safe, supervised routines are essential for meal times, moving to the hall for PE or outside for playtime, children's arrival and departure times, toileting and hand washing etc.

KEY POINT

A noisy nursery setting where staff are loud and there is constant background clatter, creates irritation and stress for both the children and staff and compromises safety.

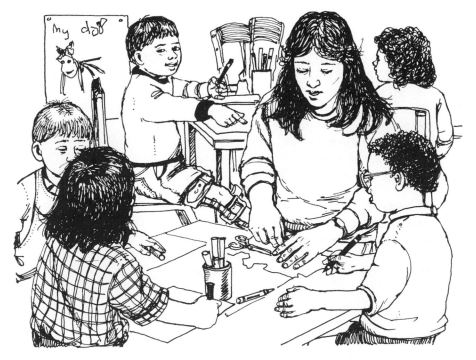

An inclusive setting welcomes children with and without special needs

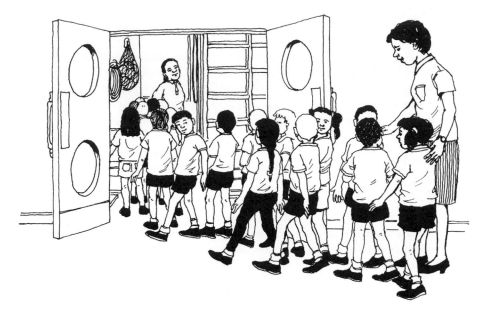

Supervising children on their way to a PE session

SAFETY CONSIDERATIONS FOR INDOOR PLAY AND LEARNING AREAS

Ventilation
All areas need ventilating regularly to:
- help prevent infection
- increase oxygen supply
- keep children and staff comfortable.

Heating
Make sure:
- heat sources are safe and adequate
- room temperatures are around 18–20°C (65–68°F).
- radiators are thermostatically controlled.

Lighting
Lighting must be safe, adequate and adjustable in order to:
- prevent eye strain
- prevent poor posture
- prevent accidents.

Furniture

Furniture should be:

- sturdy
- child-sized. There should be adjustable tables and chairs with smooth edges. All play and learning surfaces must be hygienic and the correct height for the children
- laid out to allow easy movement round it, with recognisable routes from one activity to another.

Space

Space must be sufficient for:

- floor play
- displaying children's work
- activities such as home area play, painting, sand play, water play (near water supply or sink) and woodwork
- a quiet, carpeted area for stories, reading and other calming activities, also for one-to-one time between carer and child
- safe and tidy storage of toys and materials.

Floors

Floors must be:

- even, with well-maintained non-slip coverings
- easy to vacuum and clean.

Specific safety features

Specific safety features include:

- wide entrances
- fire procedure notices (see chapter 2, page 39)
- fire exits correctly identified
- a flashing light system linked to a fire alarm
- smoke alarms
- wall mounted fire extinguishers (free standing ones can be knocked over)
- safety glass (toughened, laminated or wired) in low level (up to 76cm (2ft 6in) from floor) windows or areas of glass. Higher glass can be protected with safety film
- fitted locks on any windows that children can climb or reach up to
- the long pole for opening windows kept safely away from the children
- radiator guards
- electric socket covers
- door slam protectors
- boldly coloured arrows pointing to specific areas such as the lavatory or the playground
- safety rails along corridors.

SAFETY CONSIDERATIONS FOR OTHER SPECIFIC INDOOR AREAS

Lavatory and hand washing facilities
Requirements include:
- the recommended number of lavatory and wash basins (see chapter 2, page 43)
- child size lavatories and basins – they lessen the risk of accidents and promote independence. Long handled taps may be more suitable than the rotating type for children with poor manipulative control. A large cubicle with a lavatory and wash basin is ideal for children who may need extra help
- a thermostatically controlled hot water supply, with a temperature of around 39°C (102°F)
- lavatory partitions approximately 1.05m (3ft 6in) high
- locks on lavatory doors (if locks are used) which allow for opening from both inside and outside
- a separate room or partitioned area for nappy changing
- hand washing facilities for staff.

Hygiene measures to prevent infection are described in chapter 6, pages 140 to 152.

Rest and sleep facilities
Requirements include:
- a separate, familiar room or a partitioned area that is warm, ventilated, curtained and dimly lit
- quiet, calm conditions
- cots and stretchers spaced 44cm (18in) to 88cm (3ft) apart to allow free flow of air and lessen the risk of cross infection
- prams, cots and mattresses to recognised safety standards
- clean, aired bedding for each child (see chapter 6, page 142).

Children must always be supervised whilst sleeping, whether indoors or outdoors.

Baby and toddler nursery
Babies spend a lot of time on the floor and need plenty of space to practise rolling, crawling and walking. (See chapter 2, page 44 for desirable space standards for babies in day care.) Requirements include:
- light, airy and cheerful conditions with clean, safe floor coverings and the temperature kept around 18– 20°C (65–68°F) – check the room thermometer
- stable furniture for pulling to stand and walking round
- toys available on open shelves and interesting objects to crawl or move towards

There must be facilities for:
- preparing babies' feeds (there should be a separate milk kitchen)
- sleeping – no pillows, duvets, cot bumpers or baby nests for a child under one year (see chapter 4, page 86)

■ bathing, washing and nappy changing
■ sluicing and laundering routines.

Activities

1 From the list of specific safety features on page 109, identify those which are particularly relevant for children with special needs.
2 Look around your work setting and describe the safety features of:
  a) the windows and patio doors
  b) radiators
  c) electric sockets
  d) floor coverings
  e) children's tables and chairs.
3 Do you consider any areas of your setting to be inadequately protected? What additions might be needed to improve safety? Write up your findings.

OUTDOORS

Many children have no safe outdoor place in which to play. Not all homes have gardens. Communal play areas for children living in blocks of flats, or on housing estates, are frequently littered with dangerous debris. In addition, parents are concerned about strangers and reluctant to allow their children to play out of sight.

The playground at nursery or school may be the one place where some children can play in safety with adequate supervision. A well planned outdoor environment, with all areas visible to the carers, will offer children of different ages a wide variety of stimulating and challenging choices, freedom to run around, and opportunities for quieter moments with their friends and carers. In a nursery there should be a separate outdoor play area for babies and toddlers, preferably opening out of their play room.

New standards for playground equipment (BSEN 1176) and impact absorbing playground surfaces (see page 112) came into force on 1 January 1999. The information sheet 'The new European standards for outdoor play equipment' (available from HSE Books, PO Box 1999, Sudbury, Suffolk CO10 6FS) explains Health and Safety legislation and the role of risk assessment in the context of playground safety.

When creating an outdoor area make sure the layout is interesting and inclusive, with use made of natural ground shapes, trees and bushes. Provisions can include:

■ individual pieces of equipment such as planks, tunnels and timber structures
■ modular systems for:
  – climbing up and over
  – crawling under and through
  – swinging and balancing on
  – sliding down

- riding, pushing and pulling
■ separate spaces for:
  - wheeled toys
  - ball and group games, and for running and jumping around
  - a garden area for digging and planting activities
  - a nursery pet (for example, a rabbit run)
  - a quiet area with benches for the children to socialise with their friends
  - a sandpit.

Where space is limited, outdoor activities should be planned and offered on a rotational basis. For example, the space used for wheeled toys may be the same space used for running around and small group games.

A garden pond, being used as such, must be covered with strong netting, secured all around by a fence with a locked gate (see chapter 4, page 87) and accessible to children only with adequate adult supervision.

Accidents occur outdoors under the following conditions.
■ When supervision is poor in spite of correct staff to child ratios.
■ When equipment is:
  - poorly designed or sited
  - incorrectly installed
  - inadequately maintained
  - age and developmentally unsuitable.
■ When children wear unsuitable clothing and footwear for climbing, sliding and running. Flowing, fussy, or tight restrictive clothing, slip-on or other ill-fitting shoes and flip-flops are particularly dangerous for outdoor play.
■ When children behave inappropriately.

REMEMBER

■ Teach children to respect equipment and use it appropriately. Safety can be emphasised as you show them how to use particular items, praise their efforts and encourage them to take 'the next step'.
■ Climbing apparatus should not be used when wet and must be properly dried before children are allowed on it again.

Impact absorbing playground surfaces (IAPS)
Equipment such as swings, climbing frames, multi-tower structures and slides, and any other play equipment from which a child could fall a distance greater than 60cm (2ft), should have an impact absorbing surface (BSEN 1177) under and around it to absorb the energy of a falling child. The surface may be constructed from:
■ loose-fill material such as tree bark, or sand at least 30cm (1ft) in depth
■ 'wet pour' rubber which forms a spongy surface
■ thick rubber tiles.

Where the fall height is low (less than 60cm), grass which retains its softer top growth, is suitable, but it cannot be relied on as a safety surface when it becomes hard and dry in hot weather. Concrete, brick, stone, gravel and tarmac are not suitable surfaces. Tree bark and sand surfaces require regular inspection for raking, levelling and debris and animal fouling.

KEY POINT

Safety surfaces cannot prevent accidents, but they may reduce the seriousness of the injury. To be effective they must be suitable and well maintained.

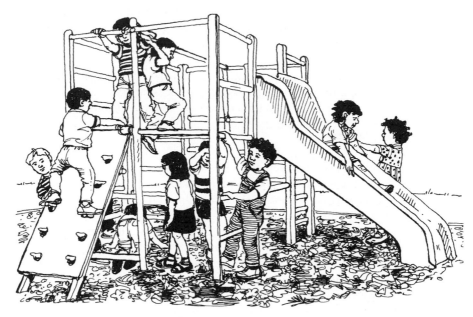

Tree bark impact absorbing surface underneath large equipment

SAFETY FOR OUTDOOR ACTIVITIES IN OUTDOOR AND PLAYGROUND AREAS

The following lists set out safety measures for outdoor activities in outdoor and playground areas. The outside area must be:
- safe
- secure
- accessible
- inclusive
- well laid out
- adequately supervised.

Playground equipment
Climbing frames, timber structures, balancing bars, slides, swings, and so on, must be:
- user-friendly, offering adventure without risk of serious accident

- well designed and to BSEN 1176 safety standard which ensures tests have been carried out for
  - stability
  - risks of trapping fingers, hand, limb or head
- well sited, for example children on swings facing the setting sun can be dazzled and become involved in collisions, or, if swings and slides are sited too closely together, children may collide as they leave them. Swings and rocking boats should be sited in isolated positions with fencing or other barrier round them
- properly installed according to manufacturer's instruction
- well maintained and serviced, and oiled as necessary
- used and supervised appropriately.

In a court action alleging negligence, reference may be made to whether equipment has met a recognised safety standard.

Outside play area

Make sure:
- ground surfaces are even and well maintained
- gates and fences are in good repair and secure
- no debris is lying around such as cans, broken glass, needles and so on
- there is no animal fouling
- no poisonous plants or trees are accessible to the children
- the sand pit is covered when not in use
- fixed equipment is safe, that bars on climbing frame are secure, nuts and screws are tightly in place and swing seats and chains are undamaged and used appropriately
- loose-fill safety surfaces are checked for depth and raked daily
- adequate and secure facilities are available for storing large and small equipment.

Children with special needs

Children with special needs must be enabled to feel part of the group and encouraged to take part in activities of their choice. A higher staff:child ratio or one-to-one key workers may be necessary to ensure adequate supervision without over protection. Some of the following additional safety measures and equipment may also be necessary:
- tricycles with pedal straps to support feet and high back rest with support belt
- bright Day-Glo strips on the edges of steps, including steps to the climbing frame and slide, and bright coloured marker lines around the swings
- hand rails along walls
- built-up edges on slides
- a slide for a child and an accompanying adult or other child
- moulded swing seats for extra support
- rails all around a trampoline.

Baby and toddler outside play area

The outside play area for babies and toddlers must be securely fenced and gated, provide plenty of space for crawling and toddling and offer shade in hot weather. A range of small-sized equipment such as climbing frames, low slides, swings and ramps, tunnels and wheeled toys, all meeting recognised safety standards, can be provided. Close supervision is essential for this age group.

The area for prams must be safe and sheltered to ensure the babies can sleep and rest in safety.

Activity

Carry out the following activity with the emphasis on safety.

a) Draw a plan of an outdoor setting for the age group of your choice (not necessarily your own setting).

b) Mark out the fences, gates and other features such as a grassed area, sand pit and quiet area.

c) Position pieces of fixed equipment and wheeled toys.

d) Write down all the safety factors you have incorporated into your plan.

STORING AND CHECKING EQUIPMENT

Storing equipment

Available storage space (often limited) must be used as economically and safely as possible, always ensuring materials and equipment can be easily accessed and moved when required.

Cupboards should not be packed so tightly that they cannot be closed and locked easily. Shelves piled high with assorted materials are a hazard. Storerooms must be kept locked and out of bounds to the children. Remember to unplug computers and televisions at the end of the day.

There are many safe storage systems.

- Low level open plan shelving and storage boxes, enable children to select toys and materials and replace them tidily on completion of an activity.
- Higher shelving should be for adult access only (as long as there is no overloading and clutter which could easily dislodge and fall on a child).
- Boxes or large drawstring bags are useful for bricks and blocks.
- Pots and jars are useful for paint brushes (thoroughly cleaned with warm water after use), drawing pencils and crayons.
- Secured boxes, cupboards or drawers are necessary for woodwork tools, sharp scissors, sewing needles, small buttons and beads and other potentially dangerous items.
- Containers with well-fitting lids should be used for dough and clay.
- There should be secure dry places for prams, wheeled toys and other moveable outdoor equipment.

Checking equipment

Nurseries and schools need plans and systems for inspecting and checking equipment and facilities. Whilst a senior member of staff will be responsible for coordinating maintenance schedules and procedures, everyone has an obligation to be involved in the safety of the setting and know to whom they must report anything damaged, malfunctioning or vandalised.

Items in need of repair should be removed, or placed out of bounds, and repaired as soon as possible. Many settings will have a caretaker or other employee whose duties might include regular inspection of the grounds, gates, fences and buildings.

Checklists or charts can be formulated for routine inspections made on a daily, weekly or termly basis. The following examples may be helpful.

On a *daily* basis, before the children arrive, check:
- the setting is generally clean and tidy
- emergency exits are unlocked and unobstructed
- the lavatory and wash room area is ready for the children – you may find a blocked wash basin, a wet floor or a damaged lavatory seat
- indoor toys and other play equipment (such as sand and water trays and home area items) are safe. Remove anything damaged or in poor condition. (These checks are often made at the end of the day when everything is cleared away, rather than in the morning.)
- doors and gates are secure and functioning properly and fences are undamaged
- playground areas for debris and animal fouling. Rake over the sand pit and loose-fill surfaces
- fixed equipment – if any item is unsafe make it out of bounds with barrier tape or immobilise in another suitable way
- timber structures for damage or splinters
- gates and doors to any basement area are locked
- pram brakes, anchor points and harnesses on prams and high chairs.

On a *weekly* basis, check:
- equipment such as fire and smoke alarms, thermostats on heating and water systems
- the amount of stored paper from children's activities (combustible material). Waste paper should be stored safely in an outside locked place until collected
- large equipment (including wheeled toys) for stability, loose nuts or bolts and so on
- rubber safety surfaces for any damage.

On a *termly* basis, check:
- indoors and outdoors thoroughly for signs of disrepair to equipment
- furnishings and fittings, paintwork, playground surfaces and outdoor seating
- rust and corrosion on iron or steel fences, gates and equipment

Many settings have an independent annual check. Make sure your checklists are completed with the following, or similar, information:

- the date of inspection
- the area and equipment inspected
- any damage or problems noted
- what action taken – immediate or further
- the signature of the person making the inspection.

REMEMBER

A checklist should not be so complicated that it is impractical to manage.

Activity

With the help of your departmental colleagues, devise a daily checklist for your setting. You can use the same formula and headings as on page 116, or arrange your own. Use the checklist each day for a week, then discuss with the group how useful and appropriate it has been. Alter it as necessary to suit the needs of your setting.

The home

A home is often referred to as 'a safe haven' but, in fact, young children, especially those under three years and those from low socio-economic groups, are very vulnerable to home accidents. Some old houses may not meet current building regulations as regards safety.

NANNIES IN THE HOME

Nannies are employed by parents to look after babies and young children in the home. It is a private arrangement with both parties agreeing terms and conditions. Nannies employed to look after the children of more than two sets of parents are required to register with the local authority.

Many of today's nannies hold a professional qualification in child care and have a certificate in, or knowledge of, First Aid practice. It is the parents' choice whether they employ a trained nanny, or a family help who may have no formal qualifications and minimal knowledge of safety and First Aid.

KEY POINT

Employers of nannies are not bound by any statutory safety law but have a duty of care, as do all citizens, towards others (including their nannies), and a civil action can be taken against them for damages to compensate for harm caused by neglect of that duty.

If you are working as a nanny, safe practice in the home must be integrated into everyday living and become an automatic part of day to day routines.

The children's bedrooms and playrooms, the stairs, kitchen, bathroom and garden are potentially dangerous areas for young children and most homes will already have some safety measures in place in these areas. However, parents may look to you for further advice and suggestions. Some safety aspects will have been discussed at your interview, others can be raised once you are in the post. It is sensible to walk around the home (indoors and outdoors) with the parents, and discuss how best to eliminate or reduce any particular hazards. For example, following your concerns, the parents may accept the necessity of safety locks on the windows in the children's rooms, or that the garden pond needs more secure fencing around it.

Hygiene and cleanliness

Whilst high standards of hygiene and cleanliness are particularly necessary in a day nursery, social cleanliness is adequate in a domestic setting once a baby is crawling around. However, bottles and teats must still be sterilised until a baby is one year old and all hygiene precautions taken with food preparation and nappy disposal and laundering. In a private home where cross infection is less likely, the use of disposable gloves for nappy changing routines is not essential.

Accident prevention measures

Many accident prevention measures set out in chapter 4, pages 75–104, apply to the home as well as day care and education settings.

The Safety Standards table in chapter 2, page 46 offers guidance on safe nursery equipment. Essential information about children's development in relation to accidents is contained in chapter 3.

In addition, and in particular, a nanny has the following responsibilities.

- To keep an up-to-date list of telephone numbers for parents' workplaces, the family doctor, health visitor, local hospital and nearest Accident and Emergency department, and the children's nursery and school numbers.
- To understand any allergy, medication or special diet a child may have.
- To check if there is a First Aid box in the home (if not, a basic one can be made up – see chapter 8, page 217).
- To find out where the gas, electricity and water mains switches are, how to turn them off, and the emergency contact numbers for these services.
- To know where keys are kept (including spare ones) for doors and windows, and check that locks and catches are easily opened (but not by children).
- To check the 'baby listening' system and night-light provision for the children's rooms and landings.
- To unplug washing machines and tumble dryers when not in use and keep the doors closed.
- To switch off and put away equipment such as food processors and blenders when not in use.
- To keep can openers, electric carving knives, razors and razor blades, scissors and glass objects out of sight and reach.

- To make sure the children's beds and other pieces of bedroom furniture are not placed in front of windows where they can be used for climbing.
- To carefully supervise the children when they are cleaning their teeth – children can poke themselves in the eye with a toothbrush or injure their throats if they fall over with a toothbrush in their mouth.
- To learn about any house pets – their behaviour patterns, routines and health care.

Useful and readily available safety equipment for the home includes:

- window locks
- multi-purpose locks for tumble dryers and washing machines
- smoke alarms
- door slam protectors
- cupboard and cabinet latches
- electric socket covers.

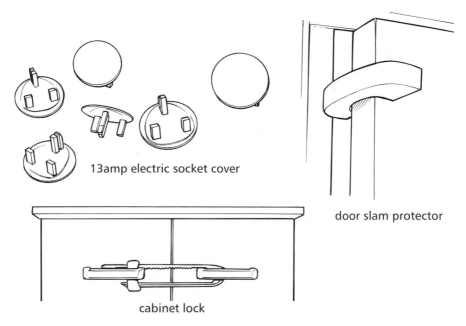

13amp electric socket cover

door slam protector

cabinet lock

Safety equipment for the home – 13amp socket cover, door slam protector and cabinet lock

Fire safety in the home

To reduce the risk of a fire in the home, all precautions set out in chapter 2, page 41 and chapter 4, pages 75–76 should be in place. You also need to ensure the following points are attended to.

- Enquire about the smoking policy in the home (adults should not smoke near the children).
- Keep cigarette lighters and matches out of sight and out of reach of the children.

- Keep children from playing too close to fires or heaters – guards must be fixed.
- Unplug all electrical equipment after use.
- Plan routes for evacuating the children from different areas of the house (for example, bedroom, playroom and kitchen) in the event of fire. Make sure the children know the ways of getting out. The home may be large and rambling, or several stories high. It may have an external fire escape, or several doors leading to the outside. If there is a child with special needs in the home, particularly a child with mobility difficulties, think about how to get her out of the house safely and quickly.
- Practice a fire drill. Make sure the children know they must shout 'fire' and get out of the house as quickly as possible
- Check where smoke alarms are sited. It may be appropriate to suggest more are installed. There should be one in the hallway and one on every floor. Check the batteries weekly.
- Never use an electric blanket in a child's bed – a covered hot water bottle, removed before the child is put down, is safer.

In the event of fire, remember the following four points.

- Shout 'fire'.
- Never stop to try and put out a fire – your priority is to get the children out, close the door and call the fire brigade. Do not stop to collect toys, comfort objects or pets.
- Get medical help if anyone is injured and then contact the children's parents.
- Do not go back inside the house until a fire officer says it is safe to do so.

KEY POINT

Chip pans are unsafe and preferably should not be used in the home with young children. Thermostatically controlled deep fat fryers are much safer.

Safety in the outside area or garden

The door to the outside area or garden should be secured so that children cannot get out unsupervised. Before the children go out to play always check the area.

- The tool shed or garage must be locked with all potentially harmful equipment and substances such as power tools, lawn mower, ladders, DIY materials, car oil, weed killer and insecticides safely inside.
- Gates and fences must be secure. Young children can very quickly dash out into the road, especially during the morning rush when you may be getting them ready for nursery or school.
- There must be no trailing or loose wires from a rotary clothes line.
- Fencing over or around the garden pond, bird bath and water butt must be secure, or the water should be emptied out (see chapter 4, page 87 for garden pond safety).
- Swings and other fixed equipment must be safe. Home made swings, or tyre swings hanging from trees must be properly secured and of adequate strength for the weight of the children.

Check there is no way a young child can get into the next door garden where there may be dangers from water sources, poisonous plants, gardening and DIY materials.

Safety for car travel and outings

Parents may agree to you taking the children out in your own car or you may have access to the family car. Make sure you follow the car safety measures described in this chapter, pages 129–132. See also 'Planning and Managing Outings', chapter 3, page 70.

Always use a harness and walking reins when taking a toddler out, especially to busy areas such as a shopping precinct, or near a main road or water.

When you feel stressed

All child care workers feel stressed in their work at some time or another. Carers in nurseries and schools can be helped by their peers and senior colleagues, but, because of the nature of their work, nannies may feel particularly isolated.

Stress may build up perhaps when a child is sick, or a toddler is going through a period of frequent temper tantrums, or perhaps a three-year-old is jealous of the new baby. Find someone to talk to and confide in – a family member or a friend or your employer. Sometimes there is a local network of nannies who can offer each other support and advice. Your doctor or the family's health visitor can also help you.

A particular source of stress may be when babies cry or they have problems with feeding. A crying, unsettled baby who is difficult to calm may arouse strong feelings of frustration, or even anger, in parents, carers or nannies. The helpful suggestions on coping with crying on page 122 are taken from the National Society for Prevention of Cruelty to Children (NSPCC) leaflet *Handle With Care*.

Whilst stress can affect both trained and untrained nannies, a qualified nanny may better understand the reasons for a baby or child's distress or behaviour, feel more confident in managing the situation, and respond more appropriately to his needs.

CHILDMINDERS

Childminders offer flexible, local, child-care services for children under eight years, for reward, in the minders' own homes. Childminders may care for:

- pre-school children during the day
- school children out of school hours and during the holidays.

The recommended childminder:child ratios are stated in chapter 2, page 44. The ratios include the childminder's own children. Parents and childminders agree the terms and conditions of individual arrangements.

The Children Act 1989 requires that childminders are registered with the local authority Social Services department. Before granting registration, the local

COPING WITH CRYING

Crying is the only way babies can tell their carers how they feel or what they need. If you've done all the obvious checks (hunger, thirst etc.) and the crying doesn't stop, try:

- cuddling the baby (remember, picking up and cuddling a crying baby isn't 'spoiling')
- gently rocking the baby in a cradle or pram
- singing
- walking up and down with the baby in your arms or in a sling
- playing music.

If the crying seems abnormal for your baby, or you think he may be unwell, consult your health visitor.

If the crying ever feels too much to bear:
Take a deep breath and let it out slowly. Put the baby down in a safe place, like a cot or pram. Go into another room and sit down for a few minutes, perhaps with a cup of tea and the TV or radio to help take your mind off the crying. Once you feel calmer, go back to your baby.
Ask a friend or relative to take over for a while.
Try not to get angry with your baby as this will only make the crying worse.
Never let things get so bad that you feel desperate. There are lots of ways you can get help. Talk to the family's health visitor or ring one of the following contacts [whose addresses are on pages 222 and 223]

SERENE (including the CRY-SIS Helpline). Offers support for parents/carers dealing with excessive crying, demanding behaviour and sleep problems.

HOME-START UK Offers support, friendship and practical help at home to families with pre-school children who are experiencing difficulties.

PARENTLINE UK Runs a network of telephone helplines for parents under stress.

NSPCC Specialises in child protection and the prevention of cruelty to children.

Reproduced with kind permission from NSPCC *Handle with Care*

authority will visit a childminder to ensure satisfactory standards of safety and home facilities are available.

- The home must be welcoming, safe and clean, with adequate space for children to rest and sleep during the day.
- Safe outdoor play space should be available.
- Sensible fire precautions must be in place such as smoke detectors, fixed guards around cooking and heating appliances, and matches locked away.

Childminders may be encouraged to undertake fire safety training. (Safe practice to prevent burn and scald accidents is detailed in chapter 4 and on pages 119–120.)

■ Good practice in hygiene routines, including nappy disposal, cleaning up body fluids (see chapter 6, pages 149–153) and food preparation (see chapter 6, pages 161–163) can be implemented.

■ High chairs, cots, buggies, bedding and potties should be available if needed. Some local authorities run an equipment loan scheme or there may be a local childminding group with similar loan arrangements.

■ The childminder should hold a First Aid Certificate, or have a knowledge of First Aid or will attend a course – local authority requirements vary.

■ Family pets should be healthy. No childminder may keep a dangerous dog.

Local authorities also have a duty to ensure that people applying to be childminders are suitable to care for children, and require applicants to have:

■ police and social services checks. (Anyone else over the age of 16 years living in the childminder's home also requires a police check.)

■ a medical check

■ satisfactory references.

Continued inclusion on the childminders' register is dependent on satisfactory visits to the home (sometimes unannounced), plus an annual inspection, by a Social Services inspector. However, this system is under review and variations in inspection and registration procedures in the United Kingdom countries are envisaged.

The relationship between parents and a childminder is one of trust and cooperation. A childminder will need to keep the following records for each child in her or his care:

■ child's name, address and date of birth

■ up-to-date home and work telephone numbers of parents/carers, family doctor and health visitor

■ emergency contact name and telephone number other than parent or carer

■ named person(s), other than parents/carers, who may collect the child

■ immunisation record

■ details of allergies, health problems and special dietary requirements

■ child's likes and dislikes

■ written permission from the parents to allow medicines or any other treatment to be given

■ particular care needs for a child with special needs.

Courses in 'Developing Childminding Practice' are available to registered childminders in England and Wales.

The National Childminding Association (address on page 222) offers a range of publications, Accident and Medication Record books, Children's Record forms and Childminding Contract forms to their members. It also coordinates childminding networks, offers free legal advice to members and maintains a national database of registered childminders.

BABY-SITTERS

There is no legal minimum age for baby-sitters. Parents are responsible for deciding the suitability of baby-sitters and judging their maturity and ability. An interview with the baby-sitter is advisable. Parents must ensure that they leave the baby-sitter a contact number plus clear and specific instructions about what to do in an emergency such as sudden illness or an accident.

Baby-sitting courses are available in some areas for young people aged fourteen to eighteen years. The course content includes basic baby and child care and establishing a good relationship with parents.

Parents may be liable in criminal law if their child is harmed whilst in the care of a baby-sitter under the age of sixteen years.

SUDDEN INFANT DEATH SYNDROME (SIDS)

Sudden Infant Death Syndrome is the sudden, unexplained death of an apparently healthy baby. It usually occurs between one week and two years of age, the peak age being two to three months. It is the commonest cause of infant death between the age of one month and one year. The incidence is higher in the winter months. A sudden infant death can occur at home, in a childminder's home, or in a nursery.

All carers of young babies need up-to-date information about SIDS and how good practice can help to reduce the risks of such a tragedy occurring among babies in their care. Factors which increase the risk of SIDS are:

■ the baby sleeping prone (on his tummy)
■ pre-term babies
■ male babies
■ multiple births
■ untreated minor ailments
■ smoky environments
■ overheating
■ socio-economic deprivation.

Role of carers in helping to prevent SIDS
■ **Place the baby supine (on his back) to sleep**, unless he has a definite medical condition for which the doctor or midwife has recommended a different position. There is no evidence of babies choking on regurgitated milk or food whilst lying on their backs.
■ **Place the baby in the *'feet to foot'* position**, that is, the baby's feet should be at

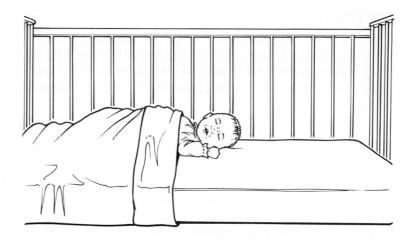

The recommended sleeping position for a baby – on her back, feet to foot of cot or pram, blankets no higher than her shoulders

the foot of the cot, with the bedclothes no higher than his shoulders. Use lightweight blankets (not duvets) and tuck them in firmly at the bottom of the cot to prevent them slipping over his head.

- **Avoid overheating**. Keep the nursery temperature about 18°C (65°F). (See also Key Points below.)
- **Ensure a smoke free environment for the baby**. Smoking during pregnancy increases the risk of SIDS, as does exposing the baby to tobacco smoke from others before and after birth.
- **Seek medical advice promptly for a baby who is unwell**, especially if he has a raised temperature, breathing problems, appears floppy or is less responsive and active than usual.
- **A baby should be taken into an adult's bed only for comfort or feeding**, then placed back in his cot to sleep
- **No one who has taken alcohol or sleeping tablets should take a baby into bed with them**. These substances will make them less alert to the baby's movements and needs.

In addition:

- encourage breast feeding
- liaise with health professionals and keep up-dated on current research into SIDS
- support families who lose a baby through SIDS.

- To prevent babies overheating do not use baby nests, duvets, pillows, cot bumpers or sheepskins or put the baby down to sleep in his cot wearing a bonnet. Babies should not sleep near radiators, heaters, fires or in direct sunlight. Remove a baby's hat and outer clothes when he comes indoors to the warmth.
- Breathing and movement monitors (not to be confused with the popular baby listening devices) are not recommended by paediatricians for 'normal' babies. They may be used occasionally under medical supervision for the benefit of specific babies.

Settle older babies down to sleep on their backs even though they will wriggle and twist. They will eventually find their own sleeping position.

Further information about SIDS can be obtained from the Foundation for the Study of Infant Deaths (FSID). The address is on page 221.

HOUSES OF MULTIPLE OCCUPANCY

You may care for children who are living long term or short term in Houses of Multiple Occupancy (HMOs) where safety standards can be poor. Hazards may include:

- unguarded stairs
- children crawling and running around in a crowded space
- worn floor coverings
- clutter on the floor and shelves
- kettle and iron used in a confined space
- overloading of electrical circuits
- old, cheap furniture which does not meet modern safety standards
- communal cooking and toilet facilities, perhaps in the basement or on a landing, which may be dirty, poorly maintained and hazardous to health
- little probability of fireproofing between the living units.

KEY POINT

Many of the above factors make the danger of fire in HMOs higher than in purpose-built flats or in homes with single family occupancy. In addition, families may prefer to use unapproved cooking facilities in their own rooms, rather than the communal facilities, so increasing the risk of burning, scalding and fire accidents.

Holidays

Nannies, in particular, are likely to care for children on holiday with the responsibility of keeping them safe and well. The following lists describe safe child care practice in preparing for a holiday, during the journey and whilst on holiday.

SAFE PRACTICE WHEN TAKING CHILDREN ON HOLIDAY

Before the holiday

Well before the holiday, you need to find out:

- whether immunisations are needed. Check with the children's doctor, and your own. Examples of immunisations are:
  - yellow fever, mainly for African countries
  - typhoid, for African and some European countries
  - hepatitis A, for Turkey, the Far East and Africa
- whether the children's tetanus immunisations are up to date
- details of the children's sleeping accommodation such as:
  - where the children will be sleeping and on which floor, whether there is a balcony, or whether a cot is provided
  - where you will be sleeping in relation to the children
- whether the drinking water is safe. If not, do you need to take water purifying tablets with you, or is boiling the water preferable? Always boil the water when preparing babies' feeds and food. Bottled mineral water is not recommended for babies and young children because of the sodium content
- what food the children are likely to be offered. If relevant, how easily can special dietary needs be met or feeds made up? Which brands of formula feed and weaning foods are available?
- the availability of medical facilities. How easily can they be accessed?
- the likely temperatures during your stay. (See chapter 4, page 84 for skin care in the sun)
- whether the beach and sea is safe for children? Does the hotel have a separate pool for young children?
- if camping or caravanning, are there any dangerous water sources nearby, such as a river, canal or lake.

Remember to pack the following:

- basic First Aid items including:
  - any current family medication
  - insect repellent, bite and sting relief
  - paediatric Paracetamol
  - antiseptic wipes and cream
  - oral rehydration sachets to prevent dehydration if a child develops diarrhoea and/or vomiting
- appropriate clothing for the country and the time of year
- an insect net for cot or pram
- sun screen and after-sun products
- necessary baby equipment and toiletries
- adequate family toiletries
- plastic shoes for wearing at the seaside – sharp shells, stones and general debris will hurt children's feet
- buoyancy aids (if paddling or swimming is on the holiday agenda).

When travelling

There are things you will need to ensure to make the journey comfortable.

- Children should have only a light meal before setting off.
- Prescribed travel sickness tablets should be taken at the recommended time.
- Clothing should be light and comfortable.
- Restraints must be checked, if travelling by car, and used at all times. Keep a car well ventilated and smoke free.
- Light snacks and drinks of water or juice (cartons are best) should be packed. Avoid juicy fruits, sticky sandwiches and chocolate.
- Potty, toilet roll, clean nappies, wipes, damp flannels, towel and disposal bags with ties should be to hand in a lidded container.
- Children should have their comfort objects, some favourite books, toys and easy to manage activities.
- Frequent breaks should be taken during the journey.
- A toddler should wear harness and reins when waiting around at an airport or on a boat.

During the holiday

Throughout the holiday be vigilant.

- Check the safety of cots, bunk beds and high chairs before using them.
- Check doors to balconies are firmly locked and secure when the children are around.
- Supervise the children carefully, especially:
  - near water (see 'Water safety and prevention of drowning', chapter 4, page 87)
  - near animals (there may be strange and unfamiliar animals in a foreign country)
  - when crossing roads, especially if driving on the right is the norm
  - in areas where there are no footpaths, roads are very busy, and traffic lights and pedestrian crossings are unfamiliar
  - in a country where poisonous plants and small animals may not be easily identified.

REMEMBER

- In areas where the drinking water supply may be unhealthy do not let the children eat ice creams, ice cubes, ice lollies or unwashed, unpeeled fruit and vegetables and make sure they clean their teeth with cooled, boiled drinking water.
- Tour operators, Embassies and Consulates can offer advice and information on the 'dos and don'ts' in particular countries.

Activity

As a nanny you are to accompany either a three-month-old baby or a two-year-old child on a holiday to Florida in August. Research the following:
a) the health and safety preparations you would need to make before the holiday and for use during the holiday
b) the clothing you would prepare for the flight and for use during the holiday.

Cars and minibuses

All road-going vehicles must, by law, have a current MOT (Ministry of Transport) Certificate of road worthiness and be appropriately taxed and insured. The law also states the following.

■ All drivers must have a licence which covers the type of vehicle they are driving.
■ Car drivers qualified with a valid full driving licence can drive a minibus with up to nine seats (including the driver's seat).
■ To drive a minibus with nine to sixteen passenger seats a driver must either:
  – a) have qualified with a valid full car driver's licence prior to 1 January 1997, or
  – b) if qualified with a valid full car driver's licence after 1 January 1997, have passed an additional test to gain a Category D1 entitlement
■ Bus and coach drivers require a PSV (Public Service Vehicle) licence.

CARS

Cars carrying young children should have childproof locks and be fitted with restraints and seat belts appropriate to the weight and physical development of the children.

Carers wishing to use their own car to transport children to and from school or nursery, or an outing, must ensure that they have insurance cover for such circumstances. Similarly, employers who allow a nanny to drive a family car must have adequate insurance cover.

Metal parts of a car seat can become very hot in sunny conditions. A heat protector placed over a child's car seat when the seat is in the car, but unoccupied, will prevent it becoming too hot. Cars can become extremely uncomfortable on hot sunny days, especially in slow moving traffic or when left parked for any length of time. To keep children comfortable:

■ dress them in loose, cotton clothing
■ make sure there is a cooling draught through the car
■ screen the windows to prevent discomfort from direct sunlight (sun blinds or screens which attach to car windows are widely available)
■ have drinks of water available.

Never leave a baby or young child alone in a car, especially in very hot weather.

MINIBUSES

All minibuses, regardless of age, must have forward facing seats with seat belts, either three point lap-and-diagonal belts or lap belts, for each child carried on an organised outing.

In a small minibus, all children must by law wear their seat belts. In larger minibuses those in the front seats must wear their belts, those in the remaining seats are strongly advised to do so. In any minibus, children under 3 years must use a child restraint (see The Law of Seat Belts, page 131), not an adult seat belt.

Children who use wheelchairs should, preferably, sit in a fixed seat during the journey and the wheelchair securely stored. Otherwise, children should be secured in their wheelchairs which are clamped to the vehicle.

Seat belts and child restraint systems

Wearing seat belts in cars became a legal requirement in 1983. Since then many lives have been saved and many people have avoided serious injury by 'belting up'. However, as many as 5,500 children are killed or injured each year whilst travelling in the back of cars. Statistics show that 70–80 per cent of parents and carers allow children to travel unrestrained in cars and that many child seats and restraints are incorrectly installed.

Carers must carefully follow the manufacturer's installation instructions. A properly installed restraint should be firm with no excessive forwards or sideways movement and the buckle of the seat belt should not rest on the frame. Look for 'Fit Safe, Sit Safe' garages – their mechanics are trained by the Child Accident Prevention Trust (CAPT).

Make sure children know that they must be correctly restrained at all times whilst travelling in the car.

KEY POINT

A child must not be in the front passenger seat if an air bag is fitted – the child restraint must be moved to the back of the car. (See page 131).

SEAT BELTS

Lap-and-diagonal seat belts are preferable to lap belts, although wearing a lap belt is far better than no belt at all. Lap belts must be secured tightly low down over the pelvic bones or top of the thighs, not over the soft stomach area. The diagonal strap of a seat belt should lie centrally over the shoulder and away from the neck. There should be no slack in whichever type of belt is worn. Never put the same seat belt around yourself and another passenger, whether adult or child.

THE LAW ON SEAT BELTS AND CHILD RESTRAINT SYSTEMS

In Law:
You **must** wear a seat belt if one is fitted. There are few exceptions to this and the driver is liable to prosecution if a child under fourteen years does not wear a seat belt.
You **must not** carry an unrestrained child in the front seat of any vehicle.
Children under 3 years travelling in the front of any vehicle **must** be carried in an appropriate restraint. The adult belt may not be used.
If an appropriate restraint is fitted in the front, but not in the rear, children under 3 years **must** use that restraint (see Key Point, page 130).
If an appropriate child restraint or seat belt is available in the front, but not in the rear, children between 3 and 11 years and under 1.5m (approximately 5ft) in height **must** use the front seat restraint or seat belt.

Reproduced by kind permission of The Stationery Office, from *Seat Belts and Child Restraints*, published by the Department of the Environment, Transport and the Regions. Crown copyright.

CHILD RESTRAINT SYSTEMS

Child restraint systems include: baby seats, child seats, booster seats and booster cushions, all of which must carry the United Nations 'E' mark or the BS Kite Mark. Child restraints are manufactured according to different weight ranges so it is the weight and physical development of a child rather than his age which determines the restraint used. Do not keep a child in a restraint once he has reached the recommended weight limit.

Some types of child restraint with the recommended weight ranges and approximate age ranges are described here.

- *Rearward facing baby seat or infant carrier* (see page 132 a)): weight range of up to 10kg (22lb), age range from birth to 9 months; or 13kg (29lb), age range from birth to 15 months. The baby is restrained by an integral (in-built) harness and the carrier secured by the adult lap-and-diagonal seat belt. This offers a high level of protection and reduces the risk of spinal cord injury in the event of an accident, but it must never be used on the front seat when a passenger airbag is fitted (see page 132). It is slightly safer to use the seat in the rear rather than the front of the car. The baby can be carried to and from the car in the seat, which may also double up as a rocking chair.
- *Forward or rearward facing child or toddler seat* (see page 132 b)): weight range of 9–18kg (20–40lb), age range of six months to four years approximately. The child is restrained by the seat's integral harness (including crotch strap to prevent the child sliding forwards) and the seat is secured by its own safety straps or by an adult seat belt.
- *Booster seat*: weight range of 9–25kg (20–55lb) with an age range of six months

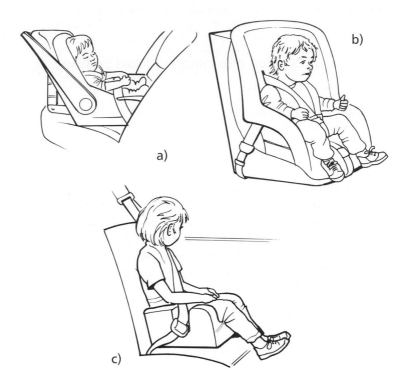

*Child restraints – a) a rearward facing baby seat or infant carrier,
b) a forward facing child or toddler seat and c) a booster cushion*

to six years. A booster seat raises the child higher and provides some sideways support. The seat and the child are restrained by the adult lap-and-diagonal seat belt which is guided through special slots. A booster seat is not designed to be used with only an adult lap belt.

■ *Booster cushion* (see c) above): weight range of 15–36kg (33–80lb), age range of four years to eleven years. Booster cushions are for children who are too large for a child seat or a booster seat. However, a young child will not have any sideways support and should preferably use a child or toddler seat. Booster cushions are used with an adult lap-and-diagonal belt. Do not use an 'ordinary' cushion instead of a booster cushion as a wriggling child may easily slip under the seat belt.

KEY POINT

It is safer for a baby to travel in an infant carrier or baby seat rather than a carrycot. A carrycot, with special restraining straps, should only be used if there is no alternative.

Air bags

Air bags are installed in many new cars. They are designed to inflate in front of the driver and front seat passenger so preventing serious head and face injuries in the event of an accident. An infant carrier or baby seat must never be used on a passenger seat fitted with an air bag. A child may be seriously injured or even killed when the bag inflates.

Safety tips

- Choose a restraint system with a recognised Safety Standard.
- Use a rear-facing baby carrier up to one year, if possible, as they offer the best protection.
- Adjust the child's harness every time the seat is used. At most, there should be only the thickness of two fingers between the harness and the child's chest. Readjust the harness if you remove a child's thick outer clothing.
- Check the car seat fitting before every journey.
- Discourage the purchase or use of a second-hand car seat – it may have been in an accident or have hidden damage.
- Always use a child's restraint in preference to an adult seat belt.
- Do not put a child in a 'higher category' restraint until he has reached the recommended weight.

Community playgrounds

A community playground is often the focal point of an outing – a safe place where children can play, socialise with their friends and enjoy using the different pieces of equipment.

Some playgrounds may have full-time formal supervision, while in others parents and carers provide a level of informal supervision as they watch their own and other children playing.

Playground providers from both the public and private sectors need to consider integrated play provision so that children with special needs are able to use the facilities should they choose to do so. Some voluntary organisations, for example the Handicapped Adventure Playground Association (HAPA), provide adventure playgrounds specifically for children with disabilities.

Ideally, community playgrounds should be carefully sited and well laid out.

- The playground should be sited on land free from hazards, with access for pedestrians (children and adults) as well as prams, pushchairs, wheelchairs and wheeled toys. The site should be overlooked so ensuring a level of community supervision.
- It should be well laid out with direct routes from one piece of equipment to another which minimise the hazards of accidental collision. All equipment must meet current safety standards. Regular maintenance and inspection procedures are essential.

DOG FOULING

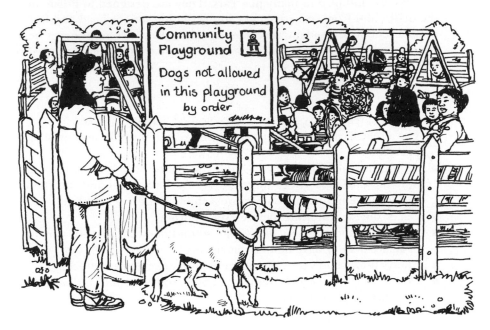

Local authorities have powers to ban dogs from community playgrounds and certain areas of public parks

Playground providers have a duty under the Environmental Protection Act 1990 to keep playgrounds and parks as clear of dog faeces as far as is practicable. Local authority control measures can include:

- fencing off a playground and installing self-closing gates to prevent dogs entering the area
- erecting clearly visible notices banning dogs from an enclosed playground
- providing 'Keep dogs on lead' notices in particular areas of a park
- providing 'Poop Scoop' notices in certain areas making it an offence for a person in charge of a dog not to remove any faeces deposited by that dog
- raising or covering a children's sand pit.

Activities

1 Look carefully at the illustration on page 135.
  a) List ten potential safety hazards for a child in this environment.
  b) How may the child be hurt by these hazards?
2 Choose five of the hazards and explain how a carer could prevent a child having an accident.

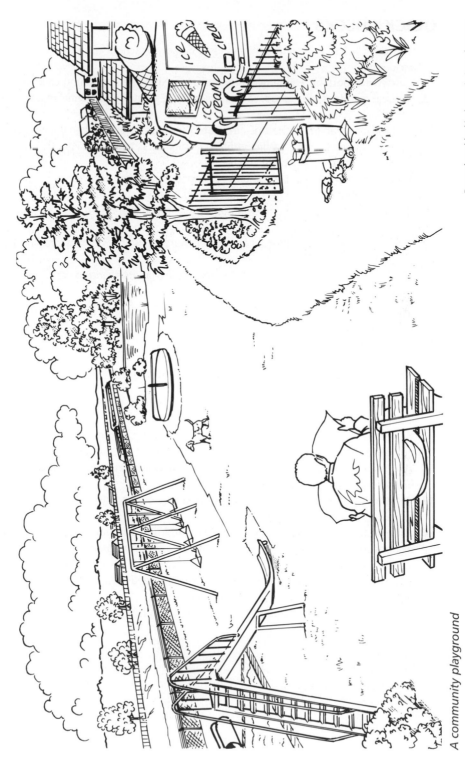

A community playground

QUICK CHECKS

1 How does lack of adequate ventilation in a nursery or school contribute to the risk of accidents?
2 State two important requirements for equipment provided for young children.
3 Give three reasons why 'good, safe and adequate' lighting is essential in a nursery or school.
4 Why must cots and stretchers be adequately spaced during children's sleep periods?
5 How would you secure a garden pond to eliminate, as far as possible, the risk of a drowning accident to a young child?
6 Name two loose-fill materials suitable as impact absorbing surfaces.
7 List several indoor safety checks which should be made by nursery staff every day.
8 List some useful safety equipment a nanny may recommend for use in a private home.
9 Why might it be more stressful for a nursery nurse to work as a nanny rather than in a nursery or school setting?
10 What helpful advice does the NSPCC offer carers who are trying to cope with a crying baby?
11 Which particular voluntary organisation offers support for parents and carers dealing with excessive crying in a baby or young child?
12 Which local authority department is currently responsible for registering childminders?
13 What three specific checks do local authorities require prospective childminders to have?
14 What are Houses of Multiple Occupancy? How might children be at risk from accidents in HM0s?
15 Which particular childhood immunisation should be up to date before a child goes on holiday?
16 Why might you need to be extra vigilant when supervising children crossing the road in a foreign country?
17 What four documents should a driver be able to produce before taking children out in a) a private car and b) a minibus?
18 a) Name the different types of car restraints. b) What is a booster cushion? c) Who is responsible for ensuring children under 14 years use appropriate restraints when travelling in a car?
19 Why must a baby carrier or child car seat never be used on a passenger seat fitted with an air bag?
20 What local authority control measures can be taken to keep dogs out of community playgrounds?

6 HEALTH AND HYGIENE

> **This chapter covers:**
> - Causes, spread and prevention of infection
> - Good hygiene practices
> - Dealing with body fluids
> - Immunity and immunisation
> - Giving medicine
> - Food hygiene
> - Pet safety and hygiene

Infection spreads rapidly when young children are grouped together, especially in overcrowded, stuffy, unventilated conditions. One child with a cold, diarrhoea and vomiting, or conjunctivitis can quickly become several, with the infection affecting both children and staff. Young children lick their fingers, cough and sneeze over others, pick their noses and forget to wash their hands – all habits which contribute to the spread of infection.

Babies are particularly vulnerable to a wide range of infections because their immune systems are immature. Children with chronic conditions such as cystic fibrosis and asthma, or those with suppressed immune systems as in leukaemia, are also at risk. Social conditions – poverty, bad housing and inadequate diet – can lead to children being less than healthy and prone to infections.

Causes, spread and prevention of infection

Micro-organisms (germs) are all around us. They live on the skin and in the nose, throat and digestive tract (stomach and bowel). They are in the air, the soil, our drinking water and milk, on the floor and on our clothes. Usually they do no harm. Some are useful, for example those living in the large bowel which help to make Vitamin K. Harmful micro-organisms, known as pathogens, cause outbreaks of common infections and other illnesses.

Professional child carers have a responsibility to help prevent the spread of infection by:
- keeping the environment clean
- attending to children's personal hygiene routines
- effective hand washing routines (children and adults)
- safe disposal of waste materials.

These routines are described in this chapter.

CAUSES OF INFECTION

The three main types of micro-organisms causing infection are bacteria, viruses and fungi.

Bacteria

Bacteria are tiny. When harmful bacteria invade the body, defence mechanisms produce antibodies which attempt to fight and destroy them. These antibodies remain ready for future use should the specific bacteria attack the body again. Bacteria can also be destroyed by antibiotics, although not all antibiotics are effective against all bacteria and occasionally the body becomes resistant to certain types of antibiotics.

Infections caused by bacteria include whooping cough, diphtheria, meningitis, tuberculosis, tonsillitis and food poisoning.

Viruses

Viruses are very much smaller than bacteria. They enter the cells of the body changing the way they work. There are no 'friendly' viruses. Although antibiotics are not effective against them, the body can produce its own antibodies against some viruses, and prevention through immunisation can be effective against others.

Infections caused by viruses include the common cold, measles, mumps, chickenpox, poliomyelitis (polio) and rubella. Meningitis and food poisoning can be viral as well as bacterial infections.

Fungi

Fungi include moulds, yeasts and mushrooms. They are simple plants which lack the green pigment, chlorophyll. Useful fungi include moulds used to make penicillin, yeasts used in bread making and alcohol fermentation, and edible mushrooms. Fungal infections include athlete's foot, ringworm, oral thrush and thrush nappy rash. Anti-fungal medicines and creams are the usual treatment. Antibiotics are generally not effective against fungal infections.

SPREAD OF INFECTION

Infections are spread by droplets in the air, via the digestive tract, by direct contact and by animals and insects.

By droplets in the air

Coughing and sneezing without covering the nose and mouth means infected droplets of moisture are carried in the air and inhaled by others. Colds, flu, measles, mumps, chickenpox and rubella are all transmitted by droplet infection.

Via the digestive tract

Food, milk or water can be infected at source, or contaminated by unhygienic preparation areas, or handlers with dirty hands. Food poisoning, in particular, is transmitted in this way.

By direct contact

Infection can pass from person to person through kissing or touching an infected person, or from using infected towels or bed linen, or sharing infected needles. Infection can also enter the body through cuts and abrasions.

By animals and insects

Animals and pets can spread illness and disease (see the table 'Some diseases transmitted by pets' on page 167). Rodents (rats and mice) and insects such as flies and cockroaches all carry germs on their bodies and can readily contaminate food. Blood-sucking types of mosquito cause malaria and yellow fever.

REMEMBER

When animal parasites (lice, worms, mites and insects) are present on the skin or inside the body it is known as *infestation*. The parasites pass easily from person to person. They are unpleasant, cause discomfort, irritation and disturbed sleep, but generally do not cause too much harm.

Signs and symptoms of infection

Clues as to the cause of an infection are provided by signs and symptoms such as a raised temperature, rash, stomach ache, diarrhoea and/or vomiting, and by laboratory investigation of samples such as blood, urine or faeces, or swabs taken from the nose or throat.

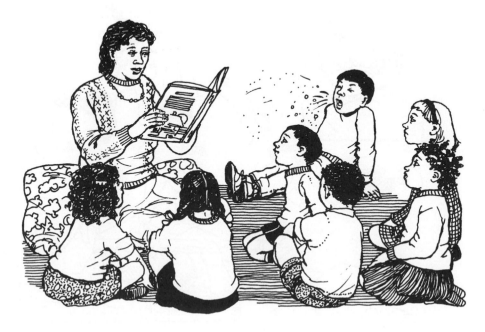

Infected droplets sprayed into the air are inhaled by others

Children with an infection should be excluded (kept away) from nursery, playgroup or school until the symptoms have cleared and they are well again. Outbreaks of infection should be reported to the area Consultant in Communicable Disease Control (CCDC). Children under five years, nursery staff and food handlers are particularly at risk from gastrointestinal infections and if there is any doubt about exclusion procedures, advice should be sought from either the CCDC or local authority Environmental Health Officer (EHO).

Activity
Check the Communicable Disease list held at your workplace. This will give details of many infections and the period of exclusion.

PREVENTION OF INFECTION

Natural defences against infection include:
- a clean, undamaged skin – it acts as a barrier against infection
- antiseptic in tears and saliva
- blood clotting – clots form a protective seal over a wound, or a tooth socket following a dental extraction, preventing blood loss and entry of infection

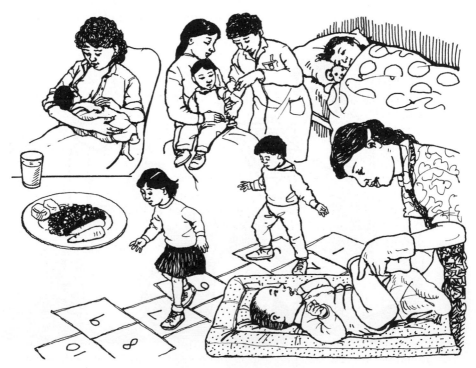

Factors which help to keep children healthy

- special acid in the stomach, white blood cells, antibodies, and useful bacteria in the bowel – all can destroy germs once they enter the body.

KEY POINT

Whilst individual resistance to infection is important, carers have a duty to enhance children's health and, as far as possible, prevent infection and illness. It is also important to involve parents as equal partners with you in child health promotion and create a climate in which you are asked for advice.

Children are less likely to be unhealthy or become ill if they:
- are breast fed in infancy
- are immunised against a range of infectious diseases
- eat a well-balanced diet – three nutritious meals and at least two healthy snacks daily. Drinks of water should always be available
- have sufficient rest and sleep and daily opportunity for outdoor play and activities. Exercise improves the circulation, stimulates the appetite, and promotes beneficial rest and sleep
- receive regular and sensitive care for their personal hygiene needs and understand the importance of hand washing (see page 148).

Public health measures such as provision of a pure, clean water supply, pasteurisation of milk and food hygiene precautions, efficient refuse collection and disposal routines, hygienic sewage disposal systems and pollution controls all play a vital role in controlling infection.

Activity

Arrange a visit to your local authority Environmental Health Department, or perhaps an Environmental Health Officer (EHO) can be invited to talk to your student group in College. Specifically, find out about:
a) the local drinking water supply – where it comes from, how it is made safe and whether fluoride is added
b) how milk is pasteurised, what happens during pasteurisation, whether there are any dangers to children from drinking untreated (green top) milk
c) the role of the EHO in inspecting food premises and his/her statutory powers to close down unsanitary businesses.
If you are unable to speak to an EHO find out the information through your own research.

Good hygiene practices

Every setting will have routines for keeping the environment clean and for attending to children's personal hygiene needs. Always follow them and understand why they are necessary.

Encourage children to look after their own health in simple ways even when they are very young. Aim to promote independence and good habits in personal hygiene by allowing children some choice in the toiletries they use, showing them what to do, helping them when necessary and praising their efforts and achievements. Always explain to children why and when they should wash their hands.

REMEMBER

Children's personal care routines should reflect the wishes of parents, including cultural practices, and take account of any special needs a child may have.

GOOD HYGIENE PRACTICE – THE ENVIRONMENT

Rooms
- Ventilate all rooms and areas thoroughly during the day. Germs flourish in warm, humid conditions.
- Vacuum and/or wash floors in nursery, play rooms and classrooms daily, damp dust furniture and ledges. Place 'wet floor' notices at the limits of wet areas.
- Vacuum carpets and upholstery daily.
- Wash paintwork and clean windows regularly.

Cots, prams and bedding
- Air cots, beds, mattresses and bedding daily.
- Launder sheets and blankets at least weekly and whenever wet or soiled.
- Clean cots, prams and beds weekly and as necessary. Babies and children newly admitted to a nursery must always have their own freshly laundered linen and newly cleaned pram, cot or bed.
- Store linen in a dry cupboard.

Lavatory and bathroom
- Keep the lavatory and bathroom area clean and dry throughout the day. Floors must be non-slip and washed daily.
- Mop up spills and 'accidents' promptly.
- Keep wash basins, taps, soap dispensers and lavatories (including seats and flush handle) clean and fresh – they all harbour germs.
- Sluice and launder towelling nappies (as on page 150).
- Thoroughly clean changing mats and potties after each use, with hot soapy water and antiseptic.
- Keep the nappy changing area clean and tidy.

Toiletries and clothes
- Keep supplies of toiletries, disposable towels, toilet tissue, face flannels, nappies, wipes, disposable aprons and gloves, and spare clothes readily available.

(In some nurseries, toiletries, nappies and spare clothes are supplied by parents for their own child.)

■ Launder soiled clothing or rinse and place in a sealed bag for the parents to take home (see page 152).

Mops and cloths

■ Thoroughly wash and bleach mops and cloths used for cleaning routines after every use and leave outside to dry – use separate colour coded ones for different cleaning routines e.g. floors, nursery furniture, cleaning up body fluids.

Hot, soapy water, at a temperature your hands can stand when wearing gloves, will clean away dirt, dust and grime but it is not hot enough to destroy all bacteria. Antiseptics, antibacterial preparations and disinfectants will kill bacteria but they do not necessarily remove dirt and grime, so just a quick wipe over surfaces and articles may not be adequate practice. Effective cleaning and hygiene routines include a *combination* of both methods.

GOOD HYGIENE PRACTICE – CHILDREN'S PERSONAL CARE ROUTINES

Routine skin care

A healthy, clear skin protects against infection. Cleaning the skin removes dirt, germs, dead skin cells, urine, faeces and vomit. Children will need variable amounts of help with hygiene routines. They usually enjoy these times of close contact and interaction with their carers, so try not to rush them. Always remain sensitive to the children's needs and the level of contact they are comfortable with. Consult with parents about any special skin care routines.

DO

- Provide a daily bath or all-over wash (especially if child is dirty, hot or sticky), or wash face and hands morning and evening and bath occasionally during the week.
- Pat skin dry, rather than rub, to prevent soreness and skin damage which could lead to infection. Take care with skin creases and between fingers and toes – black skin tends to be dry and usually needs oiling and moisturising.
- Change children's socks and underwear daily.
- Change nappies promptly whenever necessary. Never put a baby or young child down to sleep in a wet or soiled nappy.

Supplies of 'use once only' flannels in day care settings are useful for cleaning hands, faces and bottoms. Place in a bag or bin after use, ready for laundering. If cotton towels are used, children must have their own individual one, changed daily and as necessary, marked with a symbol or the child's name and kept separate from others (no less than 23cm (9in) apart), so that they do not touch when hanging on hooks. Encourage children to place disposable towels in the covered bin after use.

Routine skin care – safety

DO

- Check your personal appearance (chapter 1, page 5).
- Prepare room, equipment and clothes before bathing or washing a baby or child. Keep the room warm and the window shut.
- Check temperature of bath water with your elbow – it should feel pleasantly warm. Never add hot water once the child is in the bath. Keep the hot tap covered.
- Carefully support a young baby's head when bathing him.
- Use a non-slip safety mat in the 'big' bath.
- Use a nappy pin safely.

DO NOT

- force a child to have a bath. A frightened child can have all-over washes until he loses his fear and feels secure in the bath
- use showers for children under seven years – bursts of hot water can occur
- use talcum powder. A child may inhale the powder resulting in a choking episode or chest infection. Children with asthma and other respiratory disorders can become seriously ill
- use cotton buds to clean nose or ears, dry or moist cotton wool swabs are safer
- leave a baby or child under four years alone in the bath under any circumstances
- leave a baby alone on the changing mat.

KEY POINT

Caring for a child's skin provides you with the opportunity to observe any spots, rashes, dryness or irritation or unexplained scratches, marks or bruises which may be present. Always report and record any concerns you may have about the condition of a child's skin. (See also chapter 7, pages 170–172).

Routine hair care

Clean, well-groomed hair is a sign of good health in children. Frequency of hair washing depends largely on parental choice, but twice a week is usually adequate plus any time the hair becomes sticky and messy from day-to-day activities.

DO

- Use a non-sting shampoo, rinse the hair well in clean water and towel dry – encourage children to help with hair washing.
- Groom and dress hair according to parental wishes and cultural preference. African-Caribbean hair tends to be dry and may need oiling regularly.

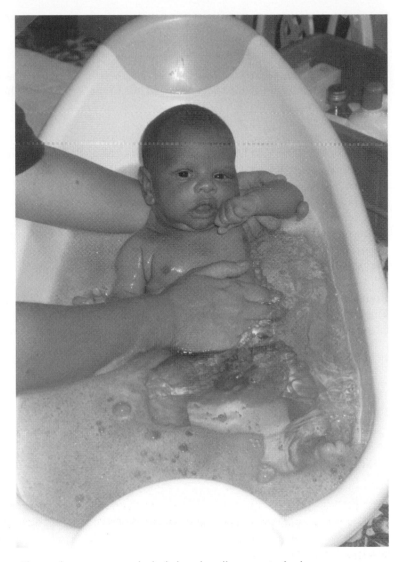

Always keep a young baby's head well supported when you are bathing him

- Allow children some choice in hair styles and accessories to promote independence and self-esteem.

- If a child dislikes hair washing keep his hair clean with a damp sponge or flannel until he loses his fear. Having a bath and hair wash with an older sibling often helps a cautious or frightened child.

- Keep children's brushes and combs separate and wash them weekly.

Routine hair care – safety

DO

- Keep shampoo out of the child's eyes – use a 'halo' guard if necessary.
- Constantly check the water temperature whilst washing the child's hair as it may vary.

Head lice

Head lice are passed on by close head-to-head contact. They do not jump or fly but simply walk from one head to another. Parents are encouraged to check their children's hair for lice and nits. Local health authorities adopt a 'rotational policy' every two to three years, informing everyone concerned which type of insecticide is currently recommended. Nurseries and schools can display leaflets or posters about head lice and the current recommended treatment. Covering the scalp with hair conditioner and wet-combing with a special detector comb can be effective treatment.

Routine nail care

Finger and toe nails need to be kept clean and trimmed to prevent dirt accumulating under them. Long finger nails can lead to scratching accidents.

DO

- Use a soft nailbrush to keep nails clean.
- Check with parents before you cut a child's nails.
- Cut nails straight across with blunt ended scissors. It is easier and safer to cut a baby's nails when he is resting or asleep.

Routine nail care – safety

DO

- Keep scissors out of children's reach.

Routine dental care

Decayed teeth cause pain, affect eating and chewing and may impede jaw development and speech. Caring for teeth in infancy and childhood helps to protect them and promote good lifetime habits.

DO

- Start dental care as soon as the first tooth appears. Use a non-fluffy cloth or babies' toothbrush and a small amount of children's toothpaste.
- Encourage and remind children to clean their teeth morning, evening and after meals. Children under eight years need help.
- Encourage regular visits to the dentist from around twelve to eighteen months.

Routine dental care – safety

DO

- Ask the pharmacist for sugar-free prescriptions. Give antibiotic medicine before meals to prevent the syrup sticking to the teeth, or follow medicine with a drink of water if the child is not eating.
- Offer children a healthy diet, avoiding sugary foods and drinks as snacks.
- Keep toothbrushes separate (bristles should not touch) and clean them in a sterilising solution weekly.
- Replace brushes every two to three months.

DO NOT

- give fluoride tablets or drops to children unless prescribed by the dentist. Fluoride is added to drinking water in some areas. Too much fluoride can damage teeth and cause staining and mottling.

Managing coughing and sneezing

DO

- Teach children to cover their nose and mouth when sneezing or coughing.
- Teach children to blow their nose instead of sniffing (this is difficult to manage under three years).
- Teach children to dispose of used tissues in a covered bin or down the lavatory. Hankies must be laundered.
- Teach children to wash their hands after blowing their nose.
- Teach children to keep tissues and hankies up sleeves or in a pocket, not to leave them lying around.
- Leave tissues within reach of the children.
- Use a cotton wool swab to clean any nasal discharge from around a baby's nose.

Managing coughing and sneezing – safety

DO NOT

- poke cotton wool, or use cotton buds, inside a baby's or child's nostrils.

Toileting

Allow children to go to the lavatory when they need to. Independence in toileting varies but, by three years, children can usually manage to pull pants and knickers down and up. Children with special needs may take longer.

DO

- Change a baby's nappy as often as necessary. Keep a record of nappy changes. Report consistently dry, or only mildly damp nappies to a senior member of staff. It may be a sign the baby is dehydrated or unwell.

- Provide individual potties, marked with the child's name or symbol.
- Respect children's privacy whilst maintaining safety and supervision.
- Help children to use toilet tissue and pull the flush. Teach girls to wipe themselves towards the flush of the lavatory, or 'from front to back'. This will prevent germs entering the bladder or vagina.
- Provide a small step for children to reach the lavatory and wash basin.
- Be alert to any abnormality of stools (diarrhoea, constipation, or blood staining) and urine (concentrated or smelly).

Toileting – safety

DO

- Provide handrails and special lavatory seats for children with special needs.
- Make sure lavatory doors can be opened from the outside.
- Restrict the numbers of children in the lavatory area at any one time.
- Make sure children wash their hands after using the lavatory.

KEY POINT

Children who are not yet toilet trained and those who wear incontinence pads will need regular care during the day to keep them fresh and dry and prevent soreness.

Activity
Plan and carry out a Dental Health Education project in your workplace to promote dental health in children.
a) Use books, puppets, games and other props to help children to understand the importance of looking after their teeth.
b) Devise a leaflet for parents and families setting out essential aspects of dental care for children, for example, the principles of a healthy diet, teeth cleaning routines, appropriate brushes and toothpaste and the use of fluoride.
c) Invite the school dentist to give a talk to the children and their parents.

HAND WASHING

One of the simplest ways to prevent the spread of infection is through hand washing. Carers and children must always wash and dry their hands :
- after using the lavatory
- after blowing their nose
- before meals or handling food
- after handling pets or pet care
- after sand or messy play.

In addition, carers must wash their hands thoroughly:
- before handling babies

- after changing a nappy
- before preparing feeds
- after giving medicines
- before (if possible) and after dealing with an accident or giving First Aid
- after cleaning up body fluids.

REMEMBER

Because of the increased use of disposable latex gloves for hygiene routines in day care settings, some carers do not understand that hands must still be washed before and after using gloves.

Hand washing will be effective if there are adequate supplies.
- There should be a warm water supply for children – around 39°C (102°F) – and a hot water supply for adults.
- A soap dispenser should be provided – it is much more hygienic than a bar of soap because it can be wiped and kept clean, and safer because soap may fall on to the floor causing a 'slipping' accident.
- Nailbrushes, kept in an antiseptic solution which is changed daily, should be available for use by carers before cleaning and sterilising feeding equipment and making up feeds, and after cleaning up body fluids.

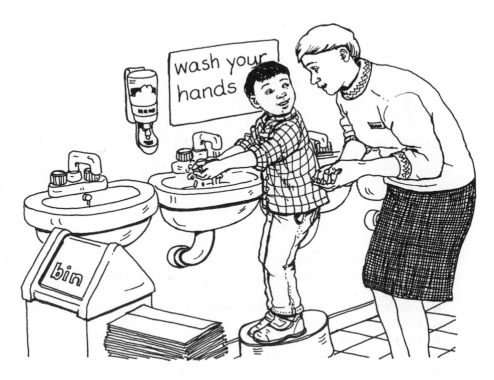

Encourage children to wash their hands correctly

- An adequate supply of disposable towels and a covered bin for disposing of them after use should be supplied. Individual, or roller, hand towels are a potential source of infection especially when they are damp from use. A hot air hand drier spreads germs around if hands are not washed properly. Also, if hands are neither washed adequately nor dried properly in the hot air, children will finish off the drying on their clothes so contaminating them.

Just splashing hands under a running tap is not an adequate hand washing routine. Always use soap, rub your palms together, wash well in between fingers and thumbs and over the backs of your hands, before rinsing well and drying with a disposable towel. Show children how to wash their hands in this way and to dispose of the used towel in the covered bin. This will encourage life-long good practice. Make sure there is a small step for children to reach the sink safely.

Activity

Create a display to help children in a nursery school or class to understand the importance of hand washing procedures.

What rhymes, stories and songs can you use, or create, to reinforce the learning in your display?

Dealing with body fluids

'Body fluids' is a term used to describe blood, urine, faeces and vomit. All settings should develop a standard procedure for dealing with body fluids.

Information and advice is available from local authority health and social services departments.

CHANGING NAPPIES

Latex disposable gloves are generally worn by nursery staff when changing babies' nappies. Wear a new pair of gloves for every nappy change. Place the used disposable nappy and gloves in a sealed bag before putting them in a lined covered bin ready for collection. Some settings have nappy disposal units.

You may care for babies who wear towelling or muslin nappies. After use place the nappies in a lidded bucket, then:

- sluice, if necessary, in a sink especially for that purpose. Remember to wear gloves
- launder using a non-biological washing powder or sanitising powder (check instructions for use)
- rinse thoroughly
- dry in the fresh air whenever possible and store in a dry place.

Always wash your hands thoroughly as soon as nappy changing is complete, clean the changing mat with hot, soapy water and antiseptic and wipe dry.

KEY POINTS

- Wearing gloves should not diminish the opportunity for interaction between the carer and child during nappy changing routines.
- Flush only the content of wet or soiled disposable nappies down the lavatory – not the whole nappy as it will create a blockage. Never leave wet or soiled nappies lying around.

Activity

Plan and carry out a hygiene routine for your early years placement, for example, hand washing, changing a nappy or bathing a baby or child. Record your routine under the following sections:

Section 1: Introduction

Include your aims and objectives for a hygiene routine a) for the baby or child and b) for the setting

Section 2: Learning outcomes

a) What do you expect to learn from this routine?

b) What do you expect the baby or child to gain from this routine?

Section 3: Planning

a) Describe how you prepared the room and equipment

b) What safety precautions did you take during preparation of the room and equipment?

Section 4: Implementation

a) Describe how you implemented this routine.

b) Comment on any unsafe situation that arose during this routine and how you reacted and intervened.

c) How did you involve the baby or child in this routine?

Section 5: Evaluation

Review this routine with special attention to the following.

a) What you learnt from this activity, including comments on areas of your own knowledge you need to develop further

b) Changes you would recommend to existing placement policy.

SPILLAGES AND SOILED ARTICLES

From time to time you will need to deal with spillages of urine, faeces and vomit as well as blood from accidents or nosebleeds. Wash any body fluid off your skin with hot water and soap. Put on disposable gloves and a protective disposable apron, then carry out the following procedures.

- If necessary, attend to the child and make him clean and comfortable.
- Absorb the spillage with paper towels and place immediately in a disposal bag.

- Using a disposable cloth, clean the soiled area with hot water and household detergent.
- Wash the area with a bleach solution made up of 1 part bleach to 10 parts cold water, or a disinfectant of the correct strength (check manufacturer's dilution instructions).
- Wash cleaning mops with a bleach solution and allow to dry outdoors.

When cleaning up carpets or other material surfaces use hot, soapy water instead of bleach.

Soiled articles should be dealt with as soon as possible using the following procedure.

- Soak blood-stained articles (towelling nappies, bedclothes or clothing) in cold water to remove the stain, before laundering in a normal washing cycle.
- Sluice articles soiled with vomit or faeces in cold water (in the special sink) before laundering in the usual way. If articles are not laundered in the setting, sluice, soak and rinse them, place in a double plastic bag, seal and label with the child's name for collection by parents.

After dealing with spillages and soiled articles, place the paper towels, cloths, gloves and apron in a double plastic bag, seal and dispose of as normal. Wash your hands thoroughly.

KEY POINT

Following all the above procedures will protect against many infections including HIV and Hepatitis B.

HUMAN IMMUNOPATHIC VIRUS – HIV

For HIV to be transmitted, the virus has to pass from an infected person into another person's bloodstream. Outside the body the virus is very fragile and is easily destroyed by exposure to air, soap, bleach and detergent. There is no known case of HIV being transmitted in a child care setting.

HIV is passed on in the following ways:

- from mother to baby either in the womb or at birth
- through breast feeding
- through sharing contaminated needles and syringes
- through unprotected sexual practices
- through infected blood or blood products.

Children can also be infected with HIV through sexual abuse.

The virus is *not* thought to be passed on in saliva, tears, sweat, urine or faeces. Nor is it transmitted by touching, hugging or shaking hands, food, coughing or sneezing, crockery or cutlery, clothes, towels, lavatory seats or door knobs.

There is no evidence that HIV is passed on in children through minor accidents such as cuts, grazes or bites. Fresh cuts bleed outwards preventing HIV getting in against the flow of blood. Clean any cuts or grazes with warm water and, if necessary, cover with a plaster or clean dressing according to your workplace practice. Show older children how to cover their own cuts with plasters or dressings and teach them not to pick up discarded litter (including needles and syringes) that could give them unnecessary cuts and grazes. See chapter 8, page 205 for care of a child with a nose bleed.

The risk of acquiring HIV in the workplace through spillage of blood, or giving First Aid to someone who is bleeding, is negligible and potential risks can be eliminated by dealing with spillages as set out in this chapter (see page 151). Always wash off any blood on your skin with soap and water as soon as possible. If blood is splashed on to your face or in your eyes, rinse with running water for a few minutes. In addition, keep your skin in good condition and cover any cuts with waterproof plasters.

Children with HIV, or Acquired Immunopathic Deficiency Syndrome (AIDS), are at greater risk of developing infections as well as serious complications from childhood infections such as measles and chickenpox. However, one of the simplest ways of protecting both children, and staff, from all infections, including HIV, is maintaining high standards of cleanliness and hygiene. In terms of hygiene and infection control, caring for all children and staff in the setting as if they had a blood borne infection will ensure good practice and equal treatment for everyone. No one will be cared for differently because of their HIV status.

HEPATITIS B

Hepatitis B is transmitted in the same way as HIV but is a more infectious disease. The immunisation programme (see 'The Department of Health current recommended immunisation programme', page 156) offers protection to babies from birth whose mothers were hepatitis B positive in pregnancy.

Immunity and immunisation

IMMUNITY

Immunity is the body's ability to resist infection. Antibodies (special blood proteins) are produced by the body in response to attack by harmful bacteria and viruses, or following immunisation. Once antibodies to a particular organism have been produced the 'fight-back' mechanism is automatically triggered when they recognise the same bacteria or viruses again. White blood cells also play a major role in fighting infection.

The three different types of immunity are natural (passive) immunity, acquired active immunity and acquired passive immunity.

Natural (passive) immunity
During pregnancy and breast feeding, a baby receives antibodies against infections which his mother has had, or been immunised against. These antibodies have mostly disappeared by the time a baby is six months old and he will need his immunisations to maintain immunity.

Acquired active immunity

Antibodies are produced as a result of either an attack of a disease or illness or immunisation. This type of immunity lasts a long time, often for many years and, with some infections, for example diphtheria, lasts for life.

Acquired passive immunity

Immunity is acquired from an injection of ready made antibodies (immunoglobulin). The protection lasts only a short time but is useful to protect an unimmunised child who has a suppressed immune system (unable to make his own antibodies) from catching an infection which could be extremely dangerous for him.

HERD IMMUNITY

When sufficient numbers of a population are immunised to prevent the spread of infection and disease it is known as 'herd immunity'. Not everybody in the population has to be immunised in order to protect a whole community, but there is a critical cut-off point. For example, in the UK, around 95 per cent of children need to be immunised against measles to prevent an outbreak of the infection and maintain immunity within the community.

In the 1940s, measles claimed 1,000 lives per year. This fell to 90 per year in the 1960s when the first measles immunisation was introduced. During the last outbreak of measles in 1980 there were 17 deaths.

Whilst parents have a right to choose whether or not to have their children immunised against a particular infection, if a sufficient number decide against immunisation then more cases of that infection will occur. This is particularly worrying for children who, for medical reasons, cannot be immunised (see 'Contra-indications to immunisation', page 155).

IMMUNISATION

Immunisation produces immunity by artificial means. When a child is immunised he receives a vaccine which contains either a very weakened dose of a specific disease, or weakened toxins (poisons) which the disease produces. This may be a 'one off' dose or the vaccine may be given over a period of a few months. The vaccines stimulate the body to produce and reproduce antibodies to particular diseases.

Immunsation is available from the family doctor or community paediatrician as part of the Child Health Promotion Programme. Most vaccines are given as an injection into the upper arm or outer thigh. The exception is the polio vaccine which is given by mouth.

All parents are offered immunisations for their children and Health Education efforts are directed towards a high uptake of immunisation. Some parents may prefer homeopathic immunisation remedies for their children instead of the Department of Health programme.

KEY POINT

Polio vaccine is excreted in the stools, so a non-immune carer of a baby recently immunised against polio is at risk of developing the disease. Strict personal hygiene, especially hand washing after nappy changing, is essential for up to six weeks after the baby's final polio vaccine dose.

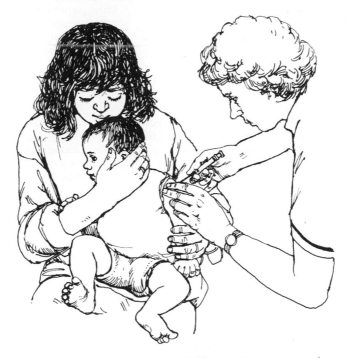

Immunisation protects young childen against a range of infectious diseases

The current Department of Health recommended immunisation programme is set out in the table on page 156.

REMEMBER

The BCG and MMR vaccines give long lasting immunity from a single injection. Three doses of Triple DTP, Polio, HIB and Group C Meningococcal vaccines given at eight, twelve and sixteen weeks are required to provide adequate immunity. Booster doses are needed of diphtheria, tetanus and polio vaccines to complete the protection, but **no** booster of pertussis (whooping cough) vaccine is required.

CONTRA-INDICATIONS TO IMMUNISATION

Children whose immune systems are impaired either because of illness or treatment (for example, treatment for some cancers) or who are HIV positive, should

The Department of Health current recommended immunisation programme

Age	Immunisation	Method	Notes
Birth	BCG (Bacille Calmette Guerin)	Injection	Given to babies: a) likely to be in contact with someone who has tuberculosis e.g.close family member b) routinely in areas where there is a large population from countries with a high incidence of tuberculosis
	Hepatitis B (1st dose)	Injection	Given to babies whose mothers were hepatitis B positive during pregnancy
4 weeks	Hepatitis B (2nd dose)	Injection	
8 weeks	Triple DTP (Diphtheria Tetanus and Pertussis, 1st dose)	Injection	One combined injection
	Polio (1st dose)	By mouth	Drops of live vaccine
	HIB (Haemophilus Influenzae Type B, 1st dose)	Injection	HIB immunisation stimulates the baby's immune system to produce antibodies against a serious type of meningitis and illnesses such as septicaemia (blood poisoning), pneumonia and epiglottitis, (inflammation of the larynx)
	Group C Meningococcal (1st dose)	Injection	A recently introduced vaccine against a type of meningitis which is one of the foremost causes of death in children and young people
12 weeks	Triple DTP (2nd dose)	Injection	
	Polio (2nd dose)	By mouth	
	HIB (2nd dose)	Injection	
	Group C Meningococcal (2nd dose)	Injection	
16 weeks	Triple DTP (3rd dose)	Injection	
	Polio (3rd dose)	By mouth	
	HIB (3rd dose)	Injection	
	Group C Meningococcal (3rd dose)	Injection	
26 weeks	Hepatitis B (3rd dose)	Injection	
12–18 months	MMR (Measles, Mumps and Rubella)	Injection	One combined injection of live vaccine. Can be given at any age after 12 months
4–5 years Earlier if starting school at 4 years	Diphtheria and Tetanus	Injection	Booster dose – one combined injection
	Polio	By mouth	Booster dose
10–14 years	Rubella	Injection	Offered only to girls if they have not already received MMR
	BCG	Injection	Offered to all pupils if tuberculin heaf test is negative
15–18 years School leavers	Diphtheria and Tetanus	Injection	Booster dose
	Polio	By mouth	Booster dose

be referred to their specialist doctor for advice as to whether or not they can be immunised.

Pertussis (whooping cough) immunisation should not be given to any child:

- following severe reaction to a previous dose
- during an acute illness
- if he has epilepsy or other neurological disorder.

Eczema or asthma, a cold or persistent runny nose or 'snuffles' on the day of immunisation *are not contra-indications to immunisations being given*.

Children with special needs should be immunised, and pre-term babies immunised according to their actual, not their expected, birth date.

POSSIBLE SIDE EFFECTS OF IMMUNISATION

Parents are particularly concerned about possible side effects from pertussis and MMR vaccines. Current medical opinion in the UK suggests that permanent harmful effects from pertussis immunisation are rare and that links between the MMR vaccine and autism and Crohn's disease (a serious bowel disorder) are unproven.

The present reduced up-take rate for MMR immunisation reflects parental concern over the vaccine. A continued low up-take level is likely to result in an epidemic of these infections (especially measles) in the next few years.

DTP (diphtheria, tetanus and pertussis) immunisation

Occasionally a baby may develop a mild fever and a small, localised red swelling over the injection site a few hours after the DTP injection. Keep the baby cool and offer him extra fluids. The symptoms should soon subside. Seek medical help, and notify the parents, if the baby has a marked raised temperature within 48 hours of the injection, is fretful and unwell, crying, vomiting, drowsy or has a convulsion. This type of reaction is rare. If the doctor decides it is a reaction to the pertussis component of the vaccine it will be omitted from future triple vaccine immunisation.

MMR (measles, mumps and rubella) immunisation

A baby may develop a mild fever and a faint bruise-like rash about a week after the injection, or some facial swelling resembling mumps around three weeks. If the baby is fretful, a recommended dose of paediatric Paracetamol can be given. Any rash or swelling will gradually subside but the baby should be seen by the doctor.

Rubella and pregnancy

Maternal rubella during pregnancy can seriously affect the unborn baby's sight, hearing, heart and brain, especially during the first two to three months. The risk of damage is less likely after about the eighteenth week. A simple blood test preconceptually will confirm a woman's immune status.

If the test is negative, immunisation will be offered with advice to avoid becoming pregnant for at least three months. Immunisation is not given if a woman is non-immune but already pregnant.

Immunisation status of carers

Carers should discuss their own immune status with their family doctor and local authority and find out whether they require immunisation against hepatitis B and rubella infections.

Activities

1 You are employed as a nanny caring for a new baby. The baby's parents are undecided about having their baby immunised. What professional advice would you give them as to the benefits of immunisation?
2 Research homeopathic immunisation available for babies and young children. How has the efficacy of homeopathic immunisation been assessed?

Giving medicine

Preferably, medicines should be given to children only if prescribed or advised by a doctor. Care should be taken with over-the-counter (OTC) medicines and used only if really necessary. Aim to promote healthy attitudes rather than reliance on medication.

Sugar-free medicines are available. Carers should be encouraged to request them when handing in a prescription. The principles of giving medicine to children are set out on page 159. Always follow them, as well as the particular guidelines and record keeping requirements of your workplace. Many settings exclude children from attending until they have finished their prescribed course of medication. This does not apply to children receiving long-term medication, for example, a child with cystic fibrosis taking daily enzyme medication or antibiotics over a prolonged period, or a child with epilepsy who may need medication during the day.

Information about giving medicines should be clear and, when necessary, available in different languages or large print, or on tape.

Since the introduction in the mid-1970s of child-resistant caps on containers the number of children attending hospital with poisoning through ingesting tablets or pills has dramatically fallen.

GIVING MEDICINE IN THE SETTING

Many settings obtain parents' written permission to give children paediatric Paracetamol when their child is unwell or has a raised temperature. In addition to this written permission, parents must always be informed when such medicine has been given to their child.

Medicine for individual children should be stored in a secure place according to the instructions. It must be clearly labelled with the child's name and directions for administration. Asthma inhalers can be kept in the nursery or school office, or First Aid room, although some children may need to keep their inhalers with them at all times for emergency use.

GIVING MEDICINES TO CHILDREN

General principles

- Written permission from parents must always be obtained before administering medicine to children.
- Medicines must be checked by two members of staff against the child's health record or prescription. Check the child's name, name of medicine, dose to be given and how often. Make sure you know what you are giving and why you are giving it.
- Use the measure provided to ensure correct dosage.
- Pour medicine with the label of the bottle uppermost, this prevents drips eventually obscuring the name and instructions.
- Always give the full prescribed course.
- After use, wipe the bottle clean with a cloth or tissue, replace the child-resistant cap and store well away from children, for example, in a fridge or locked cupboard.
- Make sure the child swallows the medicine. If a child is sick *soon* after medicine has been given, repeat the dose.
- Swallowing tablets or capsules is not easy for children. Crush them or disguise them in a little fruit juice or small piece of banana.
- Always record having given a child medicine. Nurseries and schools will have special forms but in a private home a nanny or childminder may need to make their own chart. Parents should countersign the entries when they come to collect their children.
- Throw away any medicine left after completion of the course or hand it back to the pharmacist.

REMEMBER

- Never give aspirin preparations to children, they may cause serious illness.
- Never give medicines for 'tummy aches' – the symptoms should be investigated.
- Never give medicine by mouth to a sleeping or very drowsy child, nor to a child lying down flat.
- Never give medicine prescribed for one child to any other child.
- Never give rectal suppositories without prior training and parental permission.

GIVING MEDICINE TO BABIES

Medicine prescribed for babies will be in liquid form. It must be given carefully and accurately. Do not put medicine into a baby's feed – he may refuse the feed, also the medicine can stick to the bottle and teat preventing the baby receiving the correct dose.

Food hygiene

The Food Act and Food Hygiene Regulations are set out in chapter 2, page 27.

The highest standards of hygiene are essential when storing, handling and preparing food for children. Bacteria can readily contaminate food causing food poisoning. Viruses are a less significant source of food poisoning but they cause food-related illnesses such as hepatitis A. Moulds can produce toxic substances which penetrate food, and yeasts can cause spoilage of jams and other preserves. The use of fertilisers and insecticides can also affect our food.

FOOD POISONING

Food poisoning causes diarrhoea, vomiting and abdominal pain. There may also be headache, fever and dizziness. Babies and young children can quickly become dehydrated. Always seek medical advice when a child has diarrhoea and vomiting and make sure you offer them plenty drinks of water – cooled, boiled water for babies. An outbreak of food poisoning in a nursery or school must be reported to the local authority Environmental Health Officer.

Some of the bacteria causing food poisoning
- *Bacillus cereus* – found in rice which has been kept lukewarm. Refrigeration prevents the bacteria growing.
- *Campylobacter* – found in faecal contaminated meat and poultry, and unpasteurised dairy products. Puppies and kittens, sheep and cattle can be hosts, and children can transfer this infection to their mouths when playing near infected animals. Refrigeration of food keeps it under control, cooking or pasteurisation will kill it.
- *E. coli 0157* – found in contaminated raw and undercooked meats, and unpasteurised products. It is a particular threat to young children and can lead to kidney failure and death. Bacterial growth is slowed down by refrigeration but only cooking to 70°C (150°F) or more, or pasteurisation, will kill the bacteria.
- *Listeria monocytogenes* – found in raw meat (and processed meat products) and poultry, soft cheeses, pâté, and salad ingredients. It produces flu-like symptoms, sometimes with diarrhoea. It can cause miscarriage or stillbirth, or infection in the newborn and meningitis in infants. It is resistant to refrigeration.
- *Salmonella* – found in raw and contaminated meat and poultry, raw, unwashed vegetables, and eggs. Contamination levels in eggs and chickens give cause for concern. All eggs for children must be thoroughly cooked – boiled, scrambled or poached – until both the yolk and white are hard, but they should not form part of a baby's diet until after one year. Eggs used in cakes and egg custards will be thoroughly cooked by the oven heat.

Meat and poultry, including barbecue and fast food products, must always be thoroughly cooked.

Viruses

Viruses account for many cases of diarrhoea and vomiting in babies and young children. Rotavirus infections are common in children attending nurseries. Hepatitis A infection can be spread through shellfish, water, soft fruit and, importantly, food handlers infected with the virus.

CONDITIONS FOR BACTERIAL GROWTH

Pathogens are always around waiting for the right conditions in which they can thrive and multiply. These conditions are food, moisture, warmth and time.

Food

Cooked meats and meat products, gravies and stocks, milk, eggs and products made from them, shellfish and cooked rice all attract and encourage the growth of bacteria. Some foods, however, contain additives such as salt, preservatives and acids which inhibit bacterial growth. Vacuum packaging, where oxygen has been removed, can also prevent deterioration.

Moisture

Many of the 'high risk' foods (above) contain moisture providing ideal conditions for bacterial growth. Bacteria will also multiply when fluids are added to reconstitute dried foods. The water in frozen foods (ice) is not available to the bacteria and provides safe storage, but only while the food is fully frozen.

Warmth

Blood heat is an ideal temperature for bacteria to grow. Temperatures higher than 63°C (145°F) and lower than 8°C (46.4°F) are fairly safe. Most bacteria are killed by a constant temperature of at least 70°C (158°F) that reaches to all of the food. At temperatures below 5°C (41°F), the ideal temperature for domestic fridges, bacteria do not grow and a few will die, but when food is returned to warm conditions multiplication will begin again.

Time

Bacteria grow by multiplication. In an ideal temperature they will grow by many thousands every four to five hours.

HYGIENE IN THE KITCHEN

Good personal hygiene can break the chain of infection. Hands should be kept in good condition (cracks, blemishes and broken nails all harbour germs). Antibacterial soaps and hand creams should be available and the basin for hand washing used for that purpose only and *never* for preparing food. Hand washing facilities should be available near lavatories and in the kitchen preparation area. The lavatory must not open directly into the food preparation area.

Bacteria are invisible and easily transferred from raw food to cooked food via work surfaces or kitchen utensils, or from one surface to another of used tea towels and dishcloths. Keeping the kitchen and all food preparation surfaces, sinks, equipment and utensils clean and in good working order is essential. Pets should be kept out of the kitchen.

GOOD PRACTICE IN PERSONAL HYGIENE WHEN HANDLING FOOD

DO

- Make sure a 'Wash Your Hands' notice is clearly visible in the kitchen.
- Wash hands and scrub nails thoroughly before handling food and after every interruption, especially after using the lavatory, changing a nappy, or coughing, sneezing or blowing the nose (check hand washing procedure, page 148).
- Wear clean clothing, used for food handling only. Change overalls and aprons frequently.
- Keep hair clean, tied back or covered – loose hair and dandruff contain bacteria.
- Keep nails clean and short.
- Cover the nose or mouth when sneezing or coughing.
- Dispose of tissues and hand towels into covered bins.
- Cover cuts and sores with blue waterproof dressings (easily identified if they fall off) or wear disposable gloves.
- Keep away from food preparation if infectious (with a cold, sore throat, diarrhoea, vomiting or skin infection).

DO NOT

- smoke anywhere near food
- touch the face, nose or mouth when handling and preparing food
- dip fingers into food to taste, or lick a spoon and return it to food without washing it.

ESSENTIAL KITCHEN HYGIENE

Ventilation
- There must be adequate means of natural or mechanical ventilation.
- Ventilation systems must be accessible for cleaning.

Refrigerator use
- Defrost the fridge regularly to allow it to function properly.
- Use a fridge thermometer, keep temperature about 4–5°C (39–41°F).

- Do not overload the fridge – it prevents air circulating and causes the temperature to rise.
- Cool foods before placing them in the fridge.
- Keep door-opening to a minimum.
- Store cooked food at the top, raw, uncooked food at the bottom. This prevents juices from raw food dripping onto cooked foods.
- Defrost frozen foods thoroughly.

Regular cleaning of work surfaces and floors
- Use very hot soapy water, mops, gloves and cloths for this purpose alone.
- Boil cloths and wash mops and dry them in the fresh air.

Cleaning cutlery, crockery and cooking utensils
- Dishwashers are the safest method.
- If there is no dishwasher, wear gloves, use brushes (not dishcloths) and very hot, soapy water. Rinse well in clean water, leave to drain, then clear away.
- Clean up as you go. Wipe up spills immediately.

Colour coding knives and boards for cooked or uncooked foods
- Colour code knives and boards for cooked or uncooked foods to prevent contamination, for example:
  - red labels for meat and poultry
  - blue labels for cooked meats
  - green labels for vegetables and general use.

Checking work surfaces and equipment
- To keep work surfaces and equipment in good condition check for chips, cracks and other damage.
- Ensure equipment such as mincers and can openers are easy to dismantle and are cleaned regularly and thoroughly.

Food
- Handle food as little as possible.
- Always cover food to prevent flies settling on it.
- Place food in a cool part of the kitchen or keep it in the refrigerator.
- Watch 'sell-by' and 'use-by' dates.
- Thoroughly defrost chicken and other meats before cooking – a partially cooked pink centre will be teeming with bacteria.
- When reheating previously cooked food, especially in a microwave, make sure it is thoroughly reheated until piping hot. Reheat food only once.
- Preferably, food for infants should not be stored at all.
- Foods eaten raw must be washed thoroughly.

Refuse disposal
- Remove refuse regularly from covered bins.
- Wrap waste.
- Make sure dustbins have well-fitting lids.

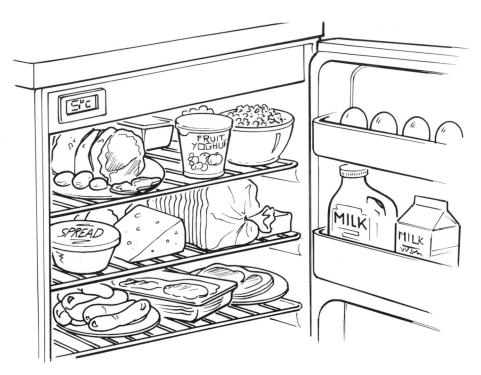

Remember to store foods correctly in a fridge

Activity

Look in your nursery or school fridge now, and check your own when you go home. If there is a fridge in the staff room, check that one as well.

a) Are the foods stored correctly, that is, cooked foods on the top shelf and raw food on the bottom shelf?
b) Are the fridges over-stocked?
c) Is there a fridge thermometer? What is the temperature? It should not be higher than 5°C (41°F).
d) When were these fridges last defrosted and cleaned?

Pet safety and hygiene

Most children love animals, especially small domestic ones. They enjoy holding and stroking them, talking to them, watching them play and grow. Many child care settings have small pets – guinea pigs, hamsters, gerbils, rabbits or fish. Whilst small caged animals present little physical danger to children they can carry diseases in their fur, feathers and faeces. New pets coming into a nursery or school setting must be checked by a vet to make sure they are healthy. Regular worming, grooming and immunisation of pets is essential to prevent them becoming unhealthy and passing on germs and disease. Children and carers must always wash their hands thoroughly after handling and caring for a pet.

The table on page 167 identifies some diseases transmitted by pets.

GOOD PRACTICE IN PET SAFETY AND HYGIENE

In a nursery or school
- A nominated person should be in overall charge of pet care and delegate the following to others:
    - feeding and general care routines
    - cleaning out the cage, hutch or tank
    - week-end and holiday care.

(Children under five years cannot manage pet care on their own.)
- If a child is allergic to a pet, remove the pet to another area of the setting.
- Keep the sandpit covered when not in use.
- Check boundary fences for damage which would allow entry to animals.

Teaching children
Teach children:
- how to care for pets
- to wear protective clothing when cleaning out or handling pets
- to wash hands thoroughly after caring for and handling a pet
- **not** to disturb sleeping pets
- **not** to tease or over excite pets
- **not** to eat pet food or allow a pet to eat from their plate
- **not** to kiss pets on the nose or mouth and never to poke a pet's eyes
- **not** to put their face near a dog or cat's mouth
- **not** to rub a pet's fur the wrong way, nor pull its tail.

Babies and young children
To avoid the risk of suffocation to babies and young children:
- use cat nets when babies are sleeping in prams outdoors
- do not let cats and dogs sleep with babies and young children – there is a danger of the pet lying over the child's face.

Emptying a litter tray or cleaning up 'a mess'
- Use gloves when emptying a litter tray, (especially important for a pregnant woman, see 'Some diseases transmitted by animals', page 167).
- If a pet makes 'a mess':
    - put on disposable gloves and apron
    - clean up with disposable kitchen towels or newspapers. Put them straight into a dustbin or burn them
    - clean the soiled area with bleach or disinfectant
    - dispose of gloves and apron safely
    - wash hands thoroughly.

Animal bite or scratch

- Wash the area of the bite or scratch with water and cover it with a clean cloth.
- Take the child to the doctor if the wound is serious or on the child's face.
- Check the child's tetanus immunity – a booster dose may be needed.

Dog owners

Owners of dogs:

- must not allow their dogs to foul pavements
- should use a 'poop scoop'
- must keep dogs out of children's play areas.

Veterinary care

Seek a vet's advice about pet care, e.g. worming and immunisations.

Always take an unhealthy or sick pet to the vet for treatment.

Activity

Write a short illustrated story about a pet of your choice for children aged three to five years. Make sure the story contains health, hygiene, caring and safety principles such as those set out on pages 164–166.

a) Read your story to the children.

b) Discuss the story with the children.

c) Evaluate how effective you were in helping them to understand the principles of pet hygiene and safety.

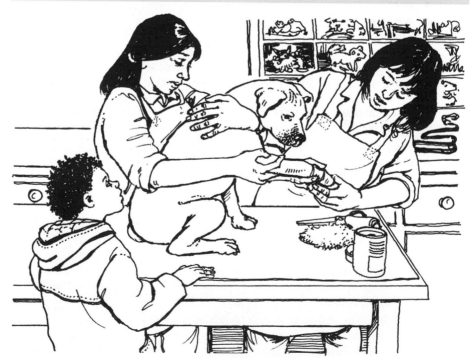

Pets must be well cared for and receive appropriate veterinary care

Some diseases transmitted by pets

Disease	Caused by	Notes
Allergies	Fur and feathers of many pets	Allergic symptoms include asthma rhinitis, dermatitis, eczema
Cat scratch fever	Cats	Can develop 3–10 days after a child has been scratched or bitten by a cat. Redness and swelling over site, fever and enlarged glands may occur
Gastroenteritis	Tortoises, terrapins, any pet who has diarrhoea	Children should not handle pets who are sick or have diarrhoea. Terrapins and tortoises should not be kept as nursery pets
Psittacosis	Birds of the parrot family, also poultry and pigeons	A viral infection inhaled from the dust and droppings in bird cages. Can cause pneumonia. Children should never feed a pet bird from their lips
Skin irritation and ringworm	Stroking or cuddling pets with fleas and mites (especially cats)	Fleas and mites are common in dogs and cats. Regular preventive grooming and shampooing is essential. Children should not handle pets with skin conditions. Nor should children with skin conditions handle pets, especially furry ones
Toxocariasis	Ingesting larvae of toxocara roundworms found in faeces of unwormed dogs and cats. The worm eggs stay in the soil long after the faeces have weathered away. Soil contamination is high in public parks	Crawling babies and toddlers playing outdoors where infected animals have fouled are at most risk. They are likely to put their fingers and playthings in their mouth and may develop toxocara infection – fever, wheezing, tummy pains, ear problems, liver damage and possibly sight loss. The infection can be controlled by making sure children wash their hands after playing in areas where dogs are allowed, after playing in soil and after handling dogs or cats. Regular worming of dogs and cats is essential.
Toxoplasmosis	Cats with diarrhoea, emptying cat litter trays, eating raw or undercooked meats	A mild infection but it can seriously harm an unborn baby. Pregnant women should wear gloves when emptying litter and avoid raw or undercooked meats

QUICK CHECKS

1 Why are babies particularly vulnerable to infection?
2 Name the three main types of micro-organisms.
3 Name three bacterial infections and three viral infections.
4 What type of infection is a) athlete's foot and b) ringworm?
5 What do you understand by the term 'droplet infection'?
6 List Public Health measures which help to prevent infection.
7 For which hygiene routines in a nursery would you wear disposable latex gloves?
8 As a carer, when *must* you wash your hands?
9 Name the three types of immunity.
10 Which immunisation vaccine is given by mouth? What potential risk does this vaccine pose to a carer?
11 What do the following abbreviations stand for: MMR, BCG, HIB?
12 Which vaccines require three doses to be given to ensure an adequate level of protection?
13 If a baby has snuffles or a cold on the day his immunisation is due, but is otherwise well, would you advise a parent to a) cancel the appointment or b) take the baby for his immunisation?
14 For which two infectious diseases should carers working with children check their own immune status?
15 What details must be shown on nursery or school children's medicine charts?
16 Name the four requirements necessary for pathogens to survive and multiply in food.
17 Which particular bacterial infection is linked to eggs and chickens?
18 Describe the personal care and hygiene precautions carers must take when handling or preparing food for children.
19 What specific allergy symptoms can the fur and feathers of pets cause?
20 Describe toxocara infection. What measures can be taken by child carers and animal owners to prevent this infection?

7 CHILD PROTECTION

> **This chapter covers:**
> ■ **Facts about child abuse**
> ■ **Identifying child abuse**
> ■ **The professional response to child abuse**
> ■ **Working with other agencies**
> ■ **Paedophilia**

Child abuse is possibly the most upsetting and demanding aspect of any child care work. Understanding when children are most at risk and from whom, can help identify and, hopefully, limit danger to children.

Facts about child abuse

While exact figures are difficult to reach, it is thought that at least one child every week is killed through abuse or neglect and that children under twelve months of age are particularly at risk. In addition, around 35,000 children are considered to be suffering or likely to suffer significant harm from their parents or carers and are on child protection registers.

Child abuse statistics cannot measure the inevitable psychological and emotional damage caused to a child in an abusive situation. Most abuse, research tells us, is committed by people whom children have most reason to trust, that is a family member or carer.

The reported numbers of children subject to abuse seem to be increasing. However, this apparent growth may be due to wider awareness of the subject, in particular that of sexual abuse. With increased knowledge, professional staff and the public are now often more willing to accept the idea that a child may be at risk and report worries and anxieties to a variety of public and voluntary bodies. The development of telephone helplines run by agencies such as the National Society for the Prevention of Cruelty to Children (NSPCC) and Child Line allow the public to express fears whilst remaining anonymous. In 1995–96, of the 60,451 referrals made through the NSPCC Child Protection Helpline, 25 per cent involved children under five years of age.

However, despite this increased awareness it is thought that only a small proportion of children who are being abused are brought to wider attention.

KEY POINT

The younger the child the more vulnerable he is, especially from physical abuse.

WHO IS LIKELY TO BE AN ABUSER?

- A parent, or cohabitant living in the home, but not related to the child, for example a step parent.
- Young unsupported parents.
- Adults who have difficulty in controlling and managing strong emotions.
- Families under stress through poverty, chronic illness, unemployment, poor housing etc.
- Parents who themselves have suffered abuse as a child.
- Parents who experienced a disruptive childhood with many changes of poor carers.

A child may be cared for by an adult who may fall into one or more of the above categories, so increasing the likelihood of abuse happening. However, it does not automatically mean that abuse will occur. The quality of the relationships the adults have together as parents, their own personalities and their own support mechanisms will all be significant in helping to prevent a repetition of an abusing cycle.

It is also is significant that abuse can take place in all economic, cultural and social groups, and can involve both men and women.

Identifying child abuse

Child abuse is any situation where a child suffers avoidable harm or is at the risk of harm by another person. This person may be a parent, a carer, or an older child. The abuse may come directly from maltreatment or provoked as a result of other problems the adult may have, for example alcohol or drug abuse, domestic violence within the home or mental health problems.

The significance of different types of injury will vary in importance depending on the age of the child. For example, bruising on the shins may be a normal part of the active development of a child through climbing, exploring, falling off bicycles etc. but not for an immobile baby of four months.

The signs and symptoms listed below do not confirm that a child has been abused but are important pointers for closer investigation. The significance is greater when several signs occur together. Since the Children Act 1989 child abuse is subdivided into separate categories, however these frequently overlap.

PHYSICAL ABUSE

Physical abuse is when a child is deliberately hurt or injured either by an adult's direct actions or by their failure to protect a child. Signs may include some or all of the following.

- Unexplained or unlikely explanations given for recent injuries.
- Failure to seek medical help following an injury.
- Fear of physical contact.
- Wearing clothing to cover injuries.

- The older child's reluctance to undress.
- Adult bite marks on the child.
- Cigarette and other burns – especially in places where an accidental brush is unlikely, for example under the arm on the body.
- Soft tissue bruising on the child – cheeks, stomach or bottom.
- Hand slap marks on the face and body. Finger grip marks around the chest in young children and babies.

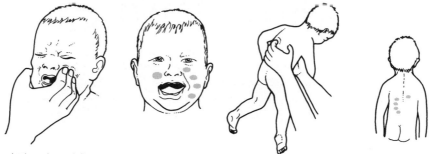

a) Thumb and finger marks on cheeks

b) Finger marks around chest

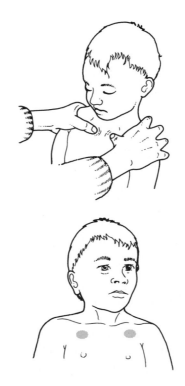

c) Thumb marks below the collar bone

Finger tip bruising

- Bruising around the mouth and damage to the frenum (under the tongue) following forced bottle feeding.
- Bleeding in the sclera – the whites of the eyes – associated in small babies with shaking.

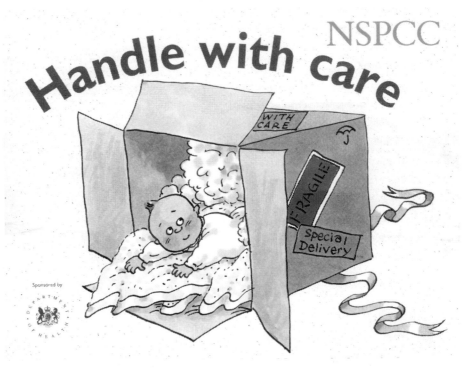

Handle with Care. Babies are fragile and precious. Never shake a baby.
Reproduced with kind permission from NSPCC

- The child showing extreme physical aggression in play with peers or is withdrawn.
- Regression in developmental progress, for example bedwetting.
- Scalds and burns in places where a reasonable explanation is unlikely, for example both soles of feet scalded equally.
- Repeated fractures and fractures with unlikely explanations, for example it is difficult to fracture a thigh bone accidentally apart from severe injury. Falling off a settee would not result in such a break. Old unreported, healed fractures that appear on X-rays.
- Signs of different stages of healing of multiple cuts and bruising.

Occasionally, inherited conditions can produce physical signs which may be mistaken for child abuse. Some birth marks, especially Mongolian spots, in children from African, Southern European and Asian backgrounds can wrongly be confused as bruises. Medical conditions such as brittle bone disease which can cause repeated bone fractures and haemophilia, the blood clotting disorder, where a child may bruise more easily, may also be mistaken for non-accidental injury.

SEXUAL ABUSE

Sexual abuse is when a child is used inappropriately for adults' sexual gratification. It does not necessarily involve actual intercourse, but could include sexual touching, masturbation, oral sex and flashing. In addition a child may be used in pornographic photographs. Signs may include some or all of the following.

- Bruising and bleeding from the genital areas, including the rectum.
- Sexually transmitted disease.
- Inappropriate and overtly affectionate behaviour from the child, especially if associated with provocative sexual approaches.
- Knowledge about sexual matters inappropriate for her age and stage of development above the normal experimental behaviour typical of nursery aged children. For example a child of four will not have experience about sexual intercourse unless she has observed, or been involved in such activity or had discussions about the subject.
- Sudden changes in behaviour and personality.
- Regression in behaviour especially bedwetting, clinging and thumb sucking.
- Difficulty in concentration, withdrawn, depression and extremes of behaviour especially in the older child, for example running away.
- Nightmares, night terrors.
- Drawing sexually explicit pictures.
- Hypersensitivity to criticism, trying to be the perfect child.
- Reluctance to undress.
- Lack of trust in known adults.
- Eating variations – food refusal or overeating, possibly weight loss and failure to thrive.

Sexual abuse may have been occurring for a long period of time and a full behavioural picture of the child will be needed for accurate conclusions to be drawn. Physical signs are not usually present in most children undergoing this type of abuse.

KEY POINT

Always listen to a child who tells you of anything that is distressing her – a young child cannot imagine sexual experiences, these must have either occurred to her or been shown to her.

EMOTIONAL ABUSE

Here, a child is continually undermined, rejected and her basic needs for love and affection are unmet. This deprivation often occurs over a long period of time. Emotional abuse is commonly associated with other aspects of maltreatment although it also stands alone. Signs may include some or all of the following.

- General developmental delay, from a baby late smiling to a school child falling behind peers in academic and social achievements.

- Physical failure to thrive – failure to gain weight and meet the norms of development expected for her age (see page 175).
- Hypersensitivity to criticism.
- Lack of confidence with a reluctance to try new experiences and challenges and a subsequent failure to develop skills and learning.
- Passivity and/or aggression.
- Speech difficulties, including delay and stammering.
- Excessive comfort type behaviour, rocking, thumb sucking, hair twisting etc.
- Emotionally needy child constantly demanding attention and affection even to strangers.

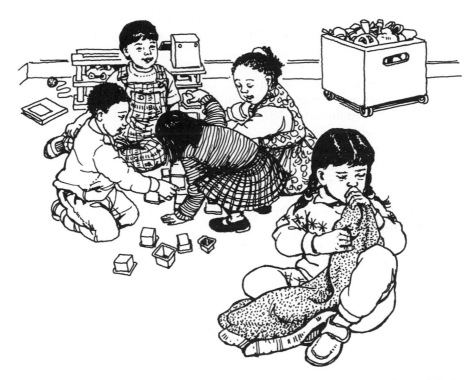

Watch for children who lack confidence, appear passive and constantly need their comfort objects

Most children at some time will display one or other of the signs of emotional distress, but a child who is abused will continue to display such signs and will also include other symptoms.

NEGLECT

Persistent or severe neglect means a parent or carer fails to provide a child with one or more of basic care, food, shelter and protection from danger. Neglect is considered abuse when it results, or is thought likely to result, in significant impairment of the child's health or development. Signs in children may include failure to thrive.

Failure to thrive

'Failure to thrive' is a term to describe babies and young children who show exceptionally poor rates of growth, usually weight but often length too. The growth measurements increasingly move from the standard rates expected for the sex and age of the child. How much an individual child should grow can be anticipated from base line measurements taken, and plotted at birth, on nationally used growth charts (see page 176). It is expected that each child will follow their own line from the point on the curve marked at birth, or move towards the average – the 50th centile. Weight, height and head circumference usually follow a similar line.

Charts are produced with standard measurements for girls and boys and for different ages.

In neglect or emotional abuse a child may show a sudden decline from their expected growth rate, or more usually a steady decline is noticed slowly ever some months.

Look at the percentile growth chart 'Girls pre-term – 52 weeks' on page 176. A girl who was born at full term weighing 3.5kg and measuring 50cm would be at the 50th centile mark. If by the time she is 40 weeks old she weighed 7kg and her length was 65cm she would have fallen to the second percentile mark and her progress would cause concern. One consideration might be she was suffering neglect or another form of abuse.

Signs of abuse

Signs of abuse in children may include some or all of the following.
- Failure to thrive, as measured on a percentile growth chart (see page 176).
- Frequently dirty, unkempt, and smelly; wears inappropriate clothing and footwear, for example cotton dresses and sandals in winter.
- Severe untreated napkin rash and cradle cap.
- Difficulty in making and maintaining social relationships.
- Erratic attendance at nursery or primary school and frequent lateness.
- Constant minor illnesses and skin rashes (these conditions are often associated with failure to seek and follow medical help).
- Hunger.
- Tiredness.
- Developmental delay.
- Destructive tendencies either in play with peers or toward herself, such as biting or scratching.

Neglect is potentially more serious for the younger child. A baby who fails to have her basic needs met is at greater physical and emotional risk as she will have few reserves on which to draw, for example, less language to ask for food and limited mobility to reach for comfort.

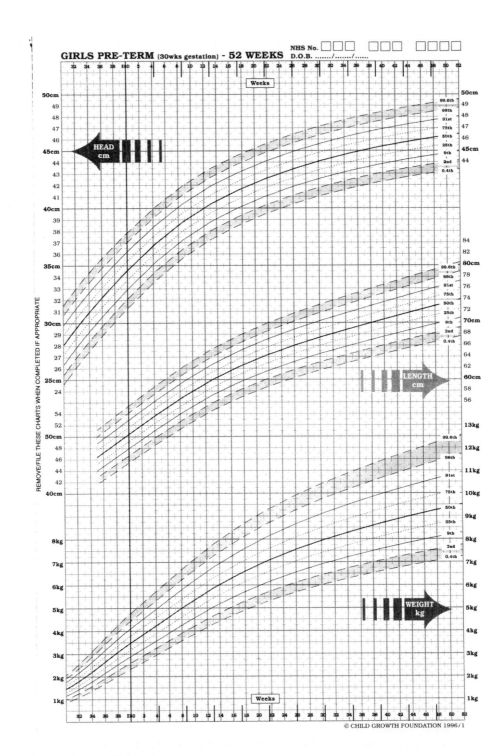

Percentile growth chart

Individual children will react to abuse in different ways and a sign that may be highly significant in one child may be less so in another. Full knowledge of a child and of child development is essential when assessing worrying behaviour or physical signs.

The professional response to child abuse

No other area of child care provokes a stronger emotional response than that of abuse, ranging from disgust, horror and anxiety, to occasionally denial, but rarely indifference. Your own background and personal experience will inevitably affect how you feel when faced with such a situation. When you are involved in working with abuse it is important to acknowledge and accept the stress this will place upon you and to use the support and advice that a nursery, or workplace provides. You should never feel you are alone if you are concerned a child may have been abused.

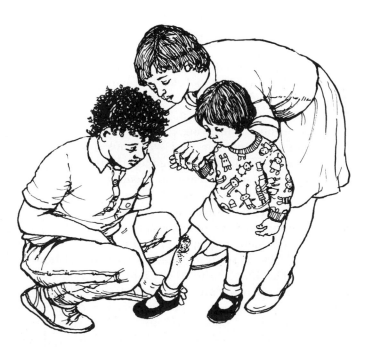

Remain open minded and non-judgemental, but always ask about injuries for which there is no obvious explanation

Make sure that what is always a distressing situation is not made worse by your response. Remain calm, professional and crucially non-judgemental. Confidentiality is essential, so gossip and chatter in inappropriate situations about issues concerned with child abuse, have no place in a professional child care worker's world. Think very carefully about with whom, and how, any information is shared. Initially, this should be only with parents, immediate workplace colleagues, and other concerned specialist professionals if the situation remains unresolved.

REMEMBER

As a professional carer your role at all times is to act to protect a child even if this is difficult or provokes controversy.

KEY POINT

The probability as to whether a child has been abused is never made following information from a single worker. You, as a carer, provide important information to help all agencies involved form a complete and accurate assessment of a child from which informed decisions, management and planning can develop.

WORK SETTING POLICIES

You must never feel isolated when faced with issues of abuse. All nurseries and schools should have current policies for managing situations when worrying signs happen that might indicate a child is at risk. Policies ensure that each situation can be professionally managed.

Policies should mean the following.

- All staff are aware of signs and symptoms indicating possible abuse. This knowledge is updated through ongoing staff training.
- All nurseries and schools have an identified staff member responsible for coordinating a response to possible abuse.
- All nurseries and schools have a working understanding of the Children Act and how it is involved in child protection.

To help develop and regulate procedures, local Area Child Protection Committees (APCPs) were developed, serving populations the size of a local authority (see 'The Role of the Area Child Protection Committee', page 179). These committees are made up of senior professionals from a wide variety of disciplines and across agencies. ACPC membership comprises workers from the social, health, education, police, and probation services, together with, usually, representatives from the NSPCC and the Racial Equality Units and other interested bodies with valid knowledge. All members are sufficiently senior to develop and implement procedures and policy.

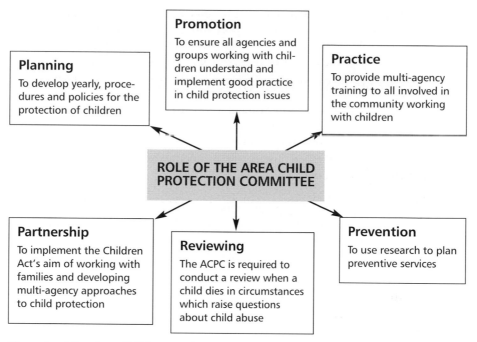

Promotion

To ensure all agencies and groups working with children understand and implement good practice in child protection issues

Planning

To develop yearly, procedures and policies for the protection of children

Practice

To provide multi-agency training to all involved in the community working with children

ROLE OF THE AREA CHILD PROTECTION COMMITTEE

Partnership

To implement the Children Act's aim of working with families and developing multi-agency approaches to child protection

Reviewing

The ACPC is required to conduct a review when a child dies in circumstances which raise questions about child abuse

Prevention

To use research to plan preventive services

The role of the Area Child Protection Committee

Activity

Find out about your local Area Child Protection Committee.
a) Who are the regular members and from what organisations and professional backgrounds are they drawn?
b) Who chairs the committee?
c) How often do they meet and where?
d) What are the local guidelines they have developed for good practice in managing child abuse in your area?

WHAT TO DO IF YOU SUSPECT SOMETHING IS WRONG WITH A CHILD IN YOUR CARE

Your response must be calm and considered. It is important to realise that you have a duty to protect any child in your care and report worrying signs to a senior member of staff even if you find this distressing.

No single carer is expected to be an expert in the management of abuse and all research tells us that good communication between the involved agencies leads to better child protection. The decision about whether abuse has or has not occurred and what will happen to the child is not yours to make alone, your role is to present facts and information and to continue your routine work with the child. This helps to increase both your own and parents' confidence in a system where no single person can draw conclusions alone and without corroboration.

Most issues of abuse are managed effectively with the child remaining in her own home but with increased support and monitoring.

THE RESPONSIBILITIES OF PROFESSIONAL WORKERS

Your responsibility as a professional worker is to know the following points.

- The policies and procedures of your workplace and what is expected of you when child abuse is suspected.
- The named member of staff responsible for management of abuse within the nursery or school.
- Where and how records should be recorded and stored.
- How to manage worrying information and with whom to share it.

When faced with a practical situation consider your response under the following headings.

- Listening to and observing the child.
- Listening to the parents.
- Reassuring the child.
- Recording all information.
- Supporting the child.

Listening to and observing the child

Always take seriously any allegations or comments a child makes. A younger child will not have the knowledge and experience to tell stories about any occurrences and if an older child feels safe and secure to disclose something painful to you, your response must be to value and respect and act on what she is saying. Never assume someone else will act on the information or notice the worrying signs.

The younger a child the fewer words she will have to indicate distress and she will need to 'tell' you in other ways. You will discover what she is trying to say through observation of her non-verbal behavioural signs, interruption to her developmental progress and possibly significant physical signs and symptoms. These observations will be helpful in providing a clear and measurable picture on which an informed decision can be reached about what may be happening to a child and if she is in danger.

A key worker should have intimate knowledge of the significance of behavioural changes in a child she has come to know well. Apparently innocent bumps and bruises may have a greater significance if viewed over a period of time and may show important patterns. Explanations of minor injuries may be revealing, for example, a child may tell you how a bruise or cut was caused or may feel somehow that she must share part of the blame for an injury – 'I was naughty so I was hit', for example.

Avoid showing revulsion or distress, whatever your own personal feelings are. The child needs you to stay calm and if you lose control it will increase her fear and insecurity.

Children with special needs are, statistically, particularly vulnerable to abuse and yet may have greater difficulty in articulating their worries, so you must observe non-verbal signs carefully.

KEY POINT

Never pump and pressurise a child to tell more than she wants. As well as frightening or distressing her she may have to repeat her story several times, which will be painful. Additionally if a disclosure results in a court hearing, it may be alleged that you have primed her and so affected the validity of the evidence.

Listening to the parents

Sharing information with parents and carers about their child and her progress, especially if you are a key worker, is routine. So, if you need explanations about apparent injuries on a child, or have worries about her behaviour ask for reasons honestly, openly and with a matter-of-fact approach. Never jump to conclusions, but remain objective and truthful in both your questions and responses. If you feel that an explanation is inadequate or information is withheld you must say that you will have to discuss the situation with a senior colleague.

Cross check any factual information given with your own records, for example dates and types of any previous injuries and reasons given from absences from nursery or school. Your response is part of a team approach and senior staff, if they remain concerned, will need to refer to social services for advice and possible action.

Inevitably, such situations are stressful and distressing, however always remember your first responsibility is to the welfare of the child.

Reassuring the child

If a child tells you something private and personal that is worrying them, and especially if a close carer or parent is involved, they need reassurance that they have behaved in the right way and that they are not to blame for any of the results. Never promise to keep any disclosure confidential but explain to the child, if she is of an age to understand, with whom you will have to share her information.

A younger child may need extra cuddles and her particular comfort objects should be at hand at difficult times. However, never force attention on a child that she does not want. Be sensitive to her particular needs at the time.

Recording all information

Always write down any information you think may be relevant to a child's safety as soon as possible – never leave recording until the next day. Use clear, accurate words, do not embellish or use subjective writing. For example saying a child appears withdrawn is subjective. You must describe her behaviour exactly – for example, 'Jane sat in the corner and refused to speak to the other children. She was sucking her comfort object and rocked for the whole two hour morning session. She was not involved in any play activities.' Or, if you consider a child is inadequately dressed for the climate describe both the temperature and what she is wearing.

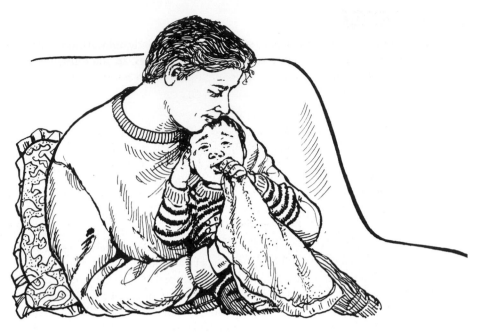

Comfort objects can help a child who is distressed

When recording physical signs – bumps and bruises – carefully describe the injury including where it is on the child's body, the size and colour and any given explanation including dates and times. It may be necessary, in some situations, for physical signs to be photographed. Senior staff will have to decide on the issues involving parental permission for such action.

Behavioural changes may need to be recorded over a period of time so ensure that dates and times are accurate.

It can be helpful both for future decision making and for your own support, to ask another colleague to observe with you and sign any observations when you complete them.

Supporting the child

This is the area of work where you will have your prime role, especially if you are the child's key worker. She needs to learn to rebuild trusting relationships with adults. Her world has been turned upside down and she needs the stability and reassurance of her daily routine, with regular attendance at nursery or school. Expect normal rules of behaviour, but offer sensitive adaptations to her routine to help her express her feelings.

Sensitive listening, encouraging her, and making time for her, as well as ensuring her physical needs are met, will be exceptionally helpful. In addition you can provide therapeutic activities to help relieve tension, soothe and release aggression in a constructive manner.

KEY POINT

Areas of intimate care such as bathing and nappy changing must always be carried out with respect for a child's privacy and cultural needs. Many settings now require male workers to have an additional adult present when performing such care routines. Always follow the policy of your setting.

Activity

1 Plan a weekly routine in which you provide activities for a three-year-old boy, James, who attends your day nursery. James has been neglected and emotionally and physically abused by his prime carers. In your plan, aim to:
   a) Release his tension and channel his aggression – use water and clay, dressing-up and role play and physical outdoor games.
   b) Promote his confidence: choose activities at which he can succeed – activities that are stretching but not causing frustration. Involve him in planning and decision making over this. Simple tasks he can do for you, like setting tables, will also boost his self-esteem.
   c) Provide extra one-to-one time: use stories, rhymes and music – select the subject matter carefully. Aim for distraction not reinforcement of distressing experiences.
   d) Check that your plan can be implemented within routine nursery attendance.

2 How might James indicate your plan had been helpful?

KEY POINTS

- While all child abuse is potentially dangerous, a child who is being physical abused is at greatest risk of death. Do not delay in seeking help if worrying physical signs appear.
- Unfortunately, a child who is experiencing other types of abuse, including sexual abuse, will have already suffered damage, which will take time and skill to manage. In these circumstances although your response must be prompt, it should not be considered a dramatic emergency and increase a child's existing anxiety. Remember, though, that categories of abuse overlap.

Working with other agencies

As soon as a suspicion of abuse appears and the policies within your local workplace have been implemented, other, multi-disciplinary agencies will become involved in investigating the allegations.

All evidence repeatedly shows that an understanding of the roles of the agencies involved in abuse, sharing of information and effective communication make decision making and subsequent action safer and more effective. The following are agencies with whose representatives you are likely to meet and work.

SOCIAL SERVICES

The local authority Social Services departments, under the Children Act are 'responsible for safeguarding and promoting the welfare of children in their area who are in need' so they have a duty to investigate possible abuse and implement the guidelines from the Area Child Protection Committee. A social worker, who may or may not already know the family, will be assigned to investigate the allegations and collect all the available information to provide a clear and accurate picture of the child and her family. She or he will interview the family including any siblings, friends, school or nursery staff and the child herself. Often a medical report is requested and this is best undertaken by a doctor the child knows well, usually the general practitioner, but occasionally a paediatrician either from the community or the hospital. All the information gathering primarily aims to include, not isolate the parents, and efforts are made to try and ensure they feel involved and part of the procedure.

In law, only Social Services departments and the Police are required to investigate allegations of child abuse or neglect. However, in the Children Act Part V, the NSPCC is named as an authorised representative able to pursue legal

---

CHILD PROTECTION ORDERS
Emergency Protection Order (EPO) This order means a child can be urgently removed to a safe place. It may be granted if the court is satisfied there is reasonable cause to believe a child is likely to suffer significant harm if she is not removed. This order is meant to be used for emergencies only and can last for eight days with a possible extension for a further seven.
Child Assessment Order (CAO) This order gives the Social Services department or the NSPCC permission for a child to be assessed to judge the extent to which she may be at risk. It is designed to be used in circumstances where there are concerns about a child's welfare but there is no hard evidence to start care proceedings or to seek an EPO. This order may be granted where a court is satisfied that there is reasonable suspicions that a child is suffering, or is likely to suffer, significant harm, and that a health or developmental assessment is necessary to establish if this is so. It is made if it is thought unlikely that the parents will agree to a satisfactory assessment unless a CAO is made. It lasts for seven days and is intended to take effect while the child is still living at home. It is not an emergency order.
Care and Supervision Order (CSO) This order places a child under the care and supervision of the local authority because she is likely to suffer, or is suffering significant harm, or not receiving reasonable care, or is beyond parental control.
Recovery Order This order is given to help recover a child who has been abducted or taken away from those who have parental responsibility for her.

proceedings and apply to the courts for any child protection orders if the parents fail to co-operate or if the child is considered to be in grave danger. These orders can be used to protect children from all types of actual abuse and risk of abuse.

THE POLICE

Specially trained child protection units are now in operation throughout the country. The Police have considerable expertise in talking to and managing children in distress as well as knowledge of the law and young people.

If the abuse is considered serious then the Police may be involved in the initial investigation, especially if there is anxiety that a criminal act has been committed or one of the legal protection orders is sought. The Police will have access to information regarding family members with records of violence involving children and of sexual offences that may be relevant to an inquiry. They will work in collaboration with Social Services and the NSPCC.

NSPCC

In parts of the country the NSPCC act as an authorised representative for Social Services (see page 184) in the initial investigation of child abuse and will collect and organise information.

HEALTH VISITORS

All families are allocated a health visitor when a baby is born. The health visitor's involvement continues until the child is at least school age, so he or she will have knowledge, not only of the child, but also the family, and will be asked for information regarding the child's medical and developmental history. The health visitor may also be asked about other relevant family information.

GENERAL PRACTITIONERS

While the GP has a code of conduct not to reveal medical information without permission, his or her prime concern is with the safety of the child and usually sees it as his or her duty to present relevant evidence if a child is seen to be at risk. Any information given will be managed in a confidential matter.

SCHOOL AND NURSERY STAFF

Key workers and class teachers will have considerable knowledge of a child to help in the development of the total picture. They should have written records, often over a period of time, which will be helpful when assessing a child.

CHILDMINDERS AND NANNIES

If a child is cared for away from the family home and her parents for long periods of time then those carers will be expected to contribute information regarding the child.

REMEMBER

Any information given to Social Services or the NSPCC must be accurate and objective, supported as far as possible with written records or other evidence.

THE CHILD PROTECTION CONFERENCE

The initial assessment over a child's welfare should be made within a maximum of seven days and if a child is considered to be in immediate danger, a legal protection order may be sought (see page 184). Usually, any action is less dramatic, information is collected and, if cause for concern remains, a Child Protection Conference, to which all involved professionals and the family are invited, is convened. This meeting should take place within 15 working days of the initial referral to Social Services or the NSPCC. The conference frequently takes place at a Social Services office but can meet in schools, nurseries or hospitals. This meeting reviews the evidence collected and makes recommendation on future action. These recommendations may range from starting legal action where the court is asked for an Emergency Protection Order (EPO) or Care and Supervision Order (CSO), placing the child on the Child Protection Register (see page 188), offering additional support for a family under stress, or no action may be thought necessary and the case will be closed.

Duties of a Child Protection Conference
- To ensure the safety and well being of the child.
- To look at all the available information, social, educational, and medical and assess if abuse has taken place.
- To consider the level of risk the child may be subject to and, if necessary, whether legal action should take place to protect the child.
- To consider possible risk to siblings.
- To consider and involve the family in decision making.

Your role at a Child Protection Conference
Your role is to contribute towards the completion of a full and accurate picture of the child about whom concerns have been expressed.

The conference will be managed by a senior child protection social worker who will introduce the participants to each other, ensure that the family members attending understand the purpose of the meeting, and will emphasise the confidential nature of the conference. The child protection social worker will ask for reports and contributions from everyone present. He or she will have a full

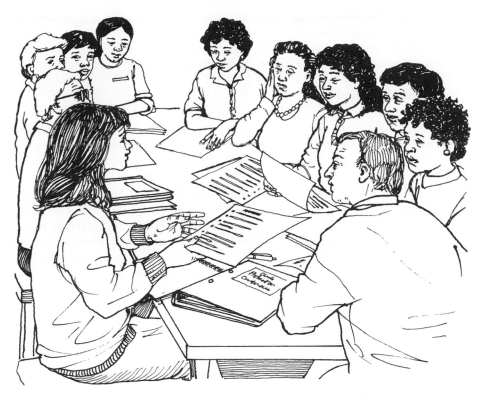

Attending a Child Protection Conference requires good preparation

knowledge and understanding of anti-discriminatory practice, and be able to look objectively at the evidence, assess the implications and summarise the findings.

A Child Protection Conference is obviously a stressful situation and you may feel anxious. However, if you have maintained a professional and honest approach with parents and carers, any information you provide should not be unexpected.

You will need to have your written reports, and observations of the child's progress with you. Always have dates, times and descriptions of any injuries, together with given explanations, carefully recorded. Support any worries you have with as much factual information as possible. Speak and contribute when requested. Remember that your special skills and expertise will be valuable, particularly your knowledge of the child, any changes you have noticed in her behaviour, any physical injuries seen, and her patterns of school or nursery attendance. This information may be known only to you and your immediate colleagues, prior to the meeting and will contribute towards completing a picture of the child.

Safe decision making depends on good communication, so always be well prepared and speak clearly using plain language, explaining any medical or technical terms you use. This will be helpful for parents and workers from other disciplines, and for those present whose first language may not be English. Be sensitive to cultural and class differences in child rearing practices and seek advice if you are unclear about issues.

Most workers will have the support of a senior colleague with them at the meeting and parents may have legal representation.

Child Protection Plan

At the conference, a Child Protection Plan will be drawn up and a key worker appointed, usually a social worker, but occasionally from another discipline, who has close and skilled knowledge of the child and her family. This key worker will be responsible for ensuring that both short- and long-term plans, agreed by the Conference to promote the child's welfare are implemented.

A key worker's duties may range from his or her preparation for any legal action to organising changes in care arrangements for the child such as increased nursery hours or after school facilities. Involvement with the family may include offering emotional support, relationship counselling and advice over housing or benefit issues. The key worker will monitor the child and her progress through regular contact with the family and liaison with other associated agencies. He or she will identify dates for calling meetings and assessing progress. All queries about the child should be directed through the key worker.

The roles of other conference members in the welfare of the child and her family will be identified, so that a cohesive approach is developed and the child's care is managed holistically.

Sometimes, the conference may conclude that having deliberated carefully on all the evidence available, no further action should be taken. Often a more formal monitoring may be thought essential and a child's name is placed on the Child Protection Register.

CHILD PROTECTION REGISTER

This is a computerised register managed and held by Social Services departments. The names of children considered to be 'at risk' are recorded, together with the alleged or proven type of abuse.

Senior officers from other agencies concerned about an individual child or family can check the Register for current information. The Keeper of the Register screens all requests for information by checking professionals' credentials and the reasons for requesting the information before it is released. Information held on the Child Protection Register include the following.

- Full name of child, including aliases or 'known names'.
- Address, sex, date of birth, ethnic and religious group.
- Full name of carer and of parental responsibility, if different.
- Details of GP.
- School, nursery or other day care centre attended.
- Date when the child was placed on the Register.
- Name and address of key worker.
- Date for review.
- Legal status of child (any court orders affecting parental rights, residency etc.).

Paedophilia

You are already aware that most child abuse occurs within a family unit. However there are individuals, outside the immediate family, who prey on children for their own sexual gratification. These people are known as paedophiles and are usually male, but sometimes can be female. They can act alone, or in local, national or even international groups. They have been known to use the Internet to spread information to other like-minded individuals. This medium can help them to infiltrate organisations where especially vulnerable children are cared for – institutions, children's groups and schools. The Internet can also be used to spread pornographic images of children around the world.

A paedophile can appear pleasant and plausible, interested in a specific child and will usually take time and effort to get to know the child, occasionally befriending the family or gaining employment in a nursery or school where the targeted child spends time. The child is often singled out for favours, special notice and praise, small gifts and non-sexual cuddling, all preparing the child to feel 'special' prior to the abuse commencing. This preparation is an attempt to gain a child's trust and to protect the abuser from the child disclosing to others – the betrayal of her particular 'friend'. Once abuse has started, children are often threatened with violence if they inform others, and can be made to believe that they instigated the abuse.

Certain children are frequently targeted by paedophiles.

- Shy, vulnerable children lacking in confidence.
- Overtly affectionate, too trusting children.
- A child already away from home, in a nursery, school or institution.
- Children with communication difficulties, especially those with disabilities.
- A child who is already suffering some type of abuse, including bullying.
- Children of a particular age, sex or racial group.

REMEMBER

- A paedophile may be a nursery worker or other child care worker.
- A paedophile will look like anyone else in the street, and will come from a wide variety of class, culture and socio-economic groups.
- A paedophile may have an important and respected position in a major organisation.

PROTECTING A CHILD FROM PAEDOPHILIA

There is a fine line between over protection and allowing a child the freedom to learn and develop. However, for a child of infant school age or under, there is some essential protection to be maintained.

- Parents and carers should always know where their child is and who is caring for her.
- The child should not be left to play unsupervised, in parks or friends' houses.
- The child should not travel on buses, trains or tubes without known escorts.

- Care must be taken in large stores and shopping malls, where the child can easily slip away.
- Reins should be used when the child is a roaming toddler in a crowded environment.
- The child's baby-sitters must be well known to the family. People advertising in newspapers and postcards in shops must not be employed without careful checking of references.
- The child must be taken to and collected from school or nursery by people in whom the parents have confidence and are of an age of responsibility.
- Nursery or school staff should not give the child into the care of adults, other than parents or carers, without written permission.
- A check by a nursery or school must be made if a parent or carer is held up and a stranger appears – even if the child recognises the adult.
- Parents and carers must always remain vigilant, observant and sensitive to a child's unexpected changes in behaviour.
- Parents and carers must always listen to a child who is old enough to tell them of any distress or anxiety.

REMEMBER

If you are concerned at any time, regarding the safety of a child, and you feel that the response of Social Services has not been satisfactory, you should always seek further advice from the Police.

Activity

1 Research the policies within your local authority for the safe collection of children from:
   a) Nursery class,
   b) Infant School,
   c) Social Services Day Care Units.
2 Is there a unified policy across all units or does each institution develop its own procedures?
3 What documentation are parents and carers asked to complete when a child is admitted to your nursery or school regarding who is allowed to collect their child?
4 What is the procedure for emergency and backup collection?
5 Do you think that a child could slip through your workplace protection net?

CENTRAL REGISTERS

The 1997 Sex Offenders Act now requires all individuals in England and Wales who have been convicted, cautioned, or who have served prison sentences for sexual offences since September 1997 to register with the Police. It is thought that 6,000 sex offenders are now registered and their names recorded.

This Act gives the Police new powers to control and restrict the movements of known paedophiles.

It is good practice for all workers in child care to undergo a police check prior to employment with children. Increasingly, police checks and disclosures of criminal records are being asked of students prior to undertaking child care training courses.

QUICK CHECKS

1 Which two agencies are required by law to investigate suspected child abuse?
2 In what situations do the Police become involved in issues of child protection?
3 Describe the four legal orders that can be used to protect children considered at risk.
4 Why might a Child Assessment Order be requested by Social Services of the Police?
5 For how long do Emergency Protection Orders and Child Assessment Orders last?
6 List five signs and symptoms that might lead you to consider a baby had been physically abused.
7 List five signs and symptoms that might lead you to consider a child of five had been sexually abused.
8 Why is it almost impossible for a child of five years to make up an allegation of sexual abuse?
9 What objective signs can indicate a toddler is suffering from neglect?
10 a) What is an Area Child Protection Committee? b) Who sits on this committee? and c) How may the expertise of this body help a local nursery?
11 Briefly, describe the four main areas of your professional responsibility, when caring for a child who may have suffered abuse.
12 You hope to open a new nursery and need to develop a Child Protection Policy. Where could you go for help with this task?
13 Why do you think effective communication is important between agencies investigating child abuse?
14 What are the tasks of a Child Protection Conference?
15 What information is included on the Child Protection Register and how is this information held and managed?
16 What is the role of the appointed key worker following a decision that a child's name should be placed on the Child Protection Register?
17 What do you understand by the term 'paedophile'?
18 List five ways a paedophile may attempt to gain a child's trust?
19 Currently, how do employers know that employees are not known sex offenders?
20 What changes are planned to increase the monitoring of convicted paedophiles?

8 FIRST AID

The earlier chapters in this book are written in order that your First Aid skills will be needed as little as possible. However, all professional child care workers must know how to cope in an emergency and when to seek extra help in situations where the prevention of an accident has failed. The information in this chapter will provide an introduction to the topic but is not intended to replace a comprehensive First Aid course.

While it is important that all staff have an understanding of First Aid, every nursery or school should have at least one worker who is the designated First Aider and known to all staff. He or she should be trained in First Aid and have completed a recognised, externally assessed course. His or her skills must be regularly updated and reassessed – at least every three years. If you are working alone in a home as a nanny or childminder, it is advisable for you, too, to undertake a recognised training course.

What is First Aid?

First Aid is the temporary treatment given in cases of accident, sudden illness or emergency, before additional medical help arrives or the child is transferred to hospital.

The aim of all First Aid is to:
- preserve life
- limit damaging effects
- help the child to recover.

Your response to any accident should be to:
- make a quick and calm assessment of the situation and, if necessary, send for help
- try to identify the nature of the injury or illness
- prioritise which treatments the child needs first and begin necessary care
- arrange transfer to hospital, surgery, or home, if needed
- keep the child comforted and comfortable and stay with him throughout treatment

- inform the parents/carers
- record the accident and your response in the accident book.

Even minor accidents which can be completely managed within the nursery, school or home will still need a full assessment.

Priorities in major emergencies

While the majority of accidents are minor, occasionally more serious incidents do happen which need prompt, confident and skilled management. A child's recovery may depend on how you act and in what order. This may be especially important if you are working alone. Focus on the immediate action needed.

OVERVIEW OF ACTION REQUIRED FOR A SERIOUS ACCIDENT

1 Review the situation and decide your immediate priorities
   ↓

2 Remove the danger
   ↓

3 Assess his response → if unconscious dial 999
   ↓

4 Maintain an airway   (A)
   ↓

5 Keep him breathing   (B)
   ↓

6 Keep his heart beating and blood circulating   (C)
   ↓

7 Check for and treat severe bleeding
   ↓

8 Treat severe burns and scalds
   ↓

9 Place an unconscious child in the recovery position and make a conscious child comfortable
   ↓

10 Seek help

---

1 REVIEW THE SITUATION AND DECIDE YOUR IMMEDIATE PRIORITIES

Remain calm and controlled. Ask any other adults to send for immediate professional help. Other children present who are not hurt, will still be frightened and they should, if possible, be taken away from the accident scene and reassured.

2 REMOVE THE DANGER

Decide if the situation is safe for you to begin First Aid. Usually immediate action is obvious, for example a fire must be put out, an electrical supply turned off, a drowning child removed from a swimming pool. Occasionally, determining on specific action may be more difficult, for example on roads. You may have to decide if it is necessary to treat a severe casualty, perhaps one with spinal injuries, in the road, as moving him might endanger his life or seriously worsen his condition. However, a road is a potentially hazardous place and you will need someone to divert and manage traffic. A difficult decision like this must be made quickly so effective First Aid can begin. It is vital, though, to remember that you will be unable to help a child if you are in danger and get hurt yourself while giving First Aid, so make sure you are safe.

3 ASSESS HIS RESPONSE

Check if he is responding – moving, crying or speaking. See if he reacts to commands to move, open his eyes or speak. Assess if he responds to painful stimuli:

- in a baby under one, flick or tap the soles of his feet
- in a child over one, place a hand on his head or body, to hold him still, then lift his arm and shake it.

If he is not responding, this means he is unconscious. Ask other adults to dial 999. Shout for help if you are alone.

BEGIN A B C

4 A = AIRWAY

As a child loses consciousness, he may vomit and the fluid may travel into his lungs, or his tongue may slip backwards over his air passage. Either of these will restrict his breathing which may become noisy, or stop. He may appear blue.

To see if the airway is obstructed, carefully remove any obvious obstruction from the front of the mouth.

- Look for his chest rising and falling.
- Listen for sounds of breathing by placing your ear close to his mouth.
- Feel for breath on your cheek.

If he is not breathing you will need to open his airway.

To open the airway in a baby:
Place the baby on his back.
Use one finger under the chin to move it forwards.
Place a hand on the back of his head and tilt the head backwards.
Look, listen and feel again for any breaths. If none are present then try artificial ventilation (see page 196).

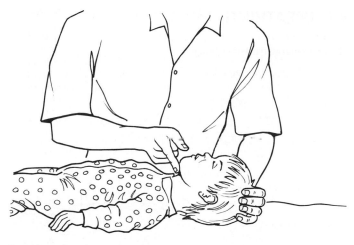
Opening the airway in a baby

To open the airway in an older child:
Place him on his back.
Place two fingers under his chin.
Place a hand on the forehead and tilt his head backwards.
Look, listen and feel again for any breaths if none are present then try artificial ventilation (see page 196).

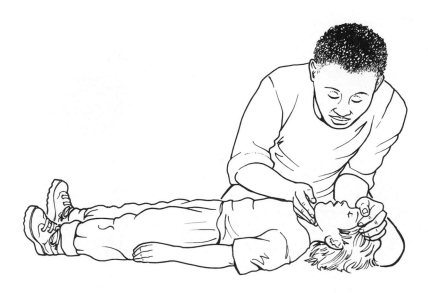
Opening the airway in an older child

5 B = BREATHING

Artificial ventilation for a baby:

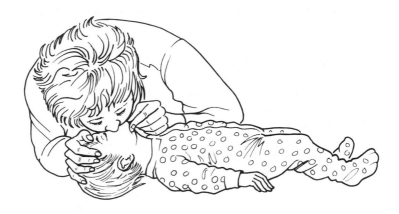

Artificial ventilation for a baby

Open the airway as on page 194.
Place your lips firmly around the mouth and nose of the baby.
Blow, gently, into the mouth and nose of the baby.
Blow at a rate of twenty breaths per minute.
After each breath, remove your mouth and watch the baby's chest fall as the air is exhaled.

Artificial ventilation for a child up to eight years:

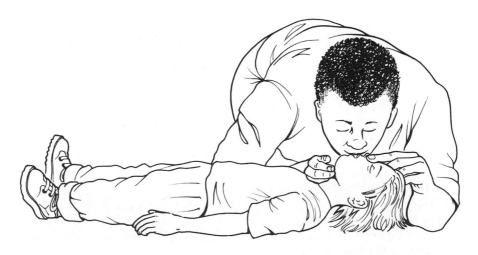

Artificial ventilation for an older child

Open the airway as on page 195.
Pinch the nostrils.
Place your lips firmly over the child's mouth.
Blow, gently, into the mouth.
Blow at a rate of twenty breaths per minute.
After each breath, remove your mouth and watch the child's chest fall as the air is exhaled.

6 C = CIRCULATION

(Keeping his heart beating and blood circulating.)
After giving the first five breaths, see if his heart is beating by checking for a pulse (remember not to use your thumb) – count for ten seconds.

Checking for a pulse in a baby:

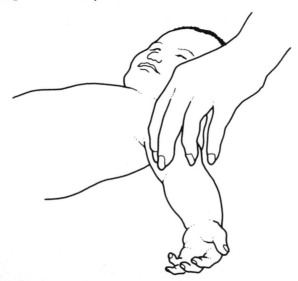

*Checking the circulation – feel the brachial pulse
on the inside of the upper arm*

Check the circulation by feeling the brachial pulse on the inside of the baby's upper arm. If you cannot detect a pulse, the heart has stopped, so start chest compression to stimulate the heart to beat.
Heart compression must be used together with artificial ventilation.

Checking for a pulse in an older child:
Feel the pulse by placing your first and second finger below the child's thumb at the wrist, or at the temple, or to the side of the windpipe.
If you cannot detect a pulse, the heart has stopped, so start chest compression to stimulate the heart to beat.
Heart compression must be used together with artificial ventilation.

Chest compression for a baby:

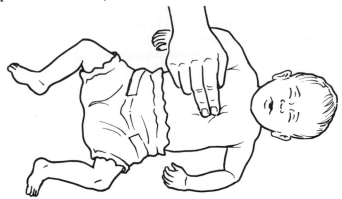

Chest compression for a baby using the tips of two fingers
Note: give five compressions per one ventilation, 100 com-
pressions per minute if working alone

Place the tips of your two fingers one finger's breadth below the baby's nipple line.
Press down sharply to a third of the depth of the chest.
Note: give five compressions per one ventilation, 100 compressions per minute if working alone.

Chest compression for a child up to eight:

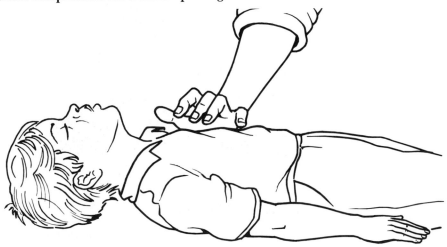

Chest compression for a child up to eight using the heel of one hand
Note: give five compressions per one ventilation, 100 compressions per minute if working alone

This is the same as for a baby but using the heel of one hand.
Note: give five compressions per one ventilation, 100 compressions per minute if working alone

KEY POINT

For chest compression use:
- the tips of two fingers for babies
- the heel of one hand for children one to eight years

Both should compress the chest to a third of its depth.
Chest compression is dangerous if the heart is beating so check for the pulse every two cycles.

Following the A B C will help you remember the order of resuscitation which you should continue until help arrives or the child shows obvious signs of recovery, then, if you can see, hear and feel his breathing, place him in the recovery position. The recovery position:
- keeps his airway open
- stops fluid – vomit or saliva – entering his lungs, with the added danger of drowning and infection.

The recovery position for a baby:

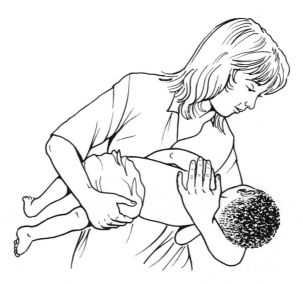

The recovery position for a baby

Hold the baby in your arms with his head tilted down to help prevent obstruction of his airways.

Recovery positions for the older child:
Place the child on his back.
1   Open the airway – see page 195.

2

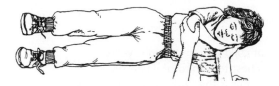

Bend the arm nearest to you at a right angle. Bring his furthest arm across his chest and cushion his cheek with the back of his hand.

3

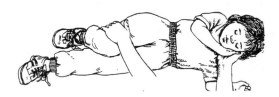

Roll him towards you. Keep his hand pressed against his cheek. Bend his outside knee, grasp him under the thigh and keeping his near leg straight, pull him towards you.

4

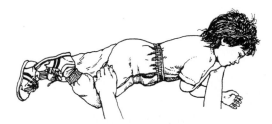

Bend his top leg at a right angle to his body to keep him on his side, and prevent him from rolling onto his front. Tilt his head back to ensure his airway remains open. Check his head is still cushioned by his hand.

7 CHECK FOR AND TREAT SEVERE BLEEDING

Stopping major fluid loss is the first priority in severe bleeding. This loss may be obvious or hidden. A child has a smaller reserve of blood than an adult, so losing even 250ml may be dangerous. If you have time, before touching any wounds, put on disposable sterile gloves.

Obvious severe bleeding
■ If the wound is clean with no signs of objects inside such as glass or metal, then apply direct pressure over the cut. Preferably, use a sterile pad and dressing, but a clean handkerchief, a towel or fingers can be used in an emergency.

Keep the pressure for at least ten minutes.

- If the wound contains sharp objects then do not apply direct pressure. Place pads either side of the wound and cover the area lightly with a sterile dressing.
- Lay the child down. If the bleeding is from an arm or leg, raise the affected limb.
- If blood soaks through the original dressing, apply another over the first.

- To reduce the risks of cross infection, routinely keep your own skin in good, clean condition, and cover any cuts with waterproof dressings.
- If you are involved in managing an accident, wash off any blood spills thoroughly, as soon as possible, using soap and hot water.

Internal bleeding
This is potentially more serious. Bleeding into joints and large internal cavities can mean that oxygen carried by the blood is diverted away from less vital organs to maintain supplies to the brain. Eventually major organs too will become affected. Shock results. Shock *must* be treated (see below).

Treating shock
In shock, the child:
- shivers
- feels faint
- has a cold, clammy skin
- has a rapid, weak pulse
- has rapid, shallow breathing
- complains of thirst.

Lay the child down and make him comfortable. If possible, raise his feet. He will be frightened, so reassure and stay with him. Keep him warm but do not overheat him as this will increase his shock.

If he complains of thirst wipe a wet tissue along his lips, but do not give him any liquid or food – he may need an anaesthetic to repair an injury. Check his pulse and breathing and record your results every ten minutes.

KEY POINT

- Shock can occur even without blood loss and can accompany accidents where there is loss of other body fluids including burns, severe diarrhoea and vomiting.
- Major pain can cause a child to become shocked.

8 TREAT SEVERE BURNS AND SCALDS

Burns can result from dry heat and corrosive substances. Scalds can result from wet heat, including hot liquids and steam. The treatment is the same.

Burns and scalds

- Stop further burning by quickly cooling the area to prevent further damage and to limit shock and pain. Gently pour cold liquid over the burn, including the face if affected, for at least 10 minutes. If an arm or a leg is burnt run the area under a flowing cold tap.
- Leave any clothing that is sticking to the wound. Burnt clothing is sterile and so should be left in place.
- Gently remove any objects that may cause constriction if swelling happens, for example rings, watches or belts, or shoe and sock if a foot is scalded.
- If possible, cover the area with a sterile dressing as burns are liable to become easily infected. If there is no sterile dressing to hand use a clean, non-fluffy tea towel or the inner sheets of plastic film. A new plastic bag is useful for a hand or foot.
- Comfort and reassure the child.
- Treat for shock (see page 201) which is likely in burns and scalds. Shock is made worse by the pain, which can be considerable, and also by fluid lost in serum oozing from burnt skin.
- Do *not*:
    - burst blisters
    - use antiseptics or medication
    - cover burns with any ointments or butter
    - use sticking plasters or adhesive dressings.

Burns to the throat or mouth

These may cause rapid swelling in the throat and close the child's airway. Look around the mouth for signs of burning on the lips, often caused by swallowing corrosive liquids which you may also smell. Never try and make him vomit.

Seek immediate urgent hospital treatment. Watch for levels of consciousness, maintain an airway and commence artificial ventilation if needed.

9 PLACE AN UNCONSCIOUS CHILD IN THE RECOVERY POSITION AND MAKE A CONSCIOUS CHILD COMFORTABLE

Ongoing care for a child who is unconscious

- Never leave a child unattended, even if he is in the recovery position.
- While awaiting help, re-check that his airway is open and he continues to breathe.
- Note his pulse and breathing rates every ten minutes and have these recorded ready to accompany him to hospital.
- Keep him warm, but do not overheat him by using hot water bottles.

Making a conscious child comfortable

A child who is involved in any accident, but especially one where blood and pain are involved, will be very frightened. He needs you to be calm. Tell him that you can help and that he will be all right. He will need his mother or father and they should be sent for immediately. While waiting, the key worker who knows the individual child best, is the most suitable person to support and comfort him until they arrive.

Other children who may have seen the accident will also be frightened. Additional members of staff should take them away from the immediate scene, then quietly explain what has happened, and involve them in routine activities. Your calm controlled manner is vital, as children will quickly become scared if they sense panic or fear in the adults.

10 SEEK HELP

Ideally, parents and carers should be the first contact if a child suffers a serious accident while in your care and every effort must be made to reach them urgently. In an emergency, the Children Act allows you to promote the child's welfare, so you could dial 999 for an ambulance or take the child to hospital without formal parental permission. In most settings, when a child is admitted, parents sign a form giving permission for emergency treatment. This will be stored with the standard health records, and these also should be ready to accompany the child to hospital (see page 218).

Information should be kept by the telephone for emergency access and must include:

- the name, address and telephone number of the nearest hospital Accident and Emergency department
- the exact address and location of the unit to give to emergency services.

Additional information will be needed by the hospital and will include:

- how, when and where the accident happened
- timings – especially important if the child lost consciousness
- any First Aid measures undertaken
- careful descriptions of specific signs and symptoms, for example, in blood loss, what amount and whether blood was pumping or seeping out.

Recording the accident

As soon as it is possible write a full, accurate, account of the accident in the accident book (see page 218). A senior staff member should read and countersign the record. In a serious accident, additional reports from other involved workers may be needed. If you are working in a private home you should still fully document the facts of the accident, in writing, while your memory is fresh. A copy of the report should be given to the parents or carer.

Accounting for a major accident enables:

- staff to reflect on practice and see whether changes are necessary, or lessons are to be learnt
- planning for any staff training and updating of skills that have been identified as necessary.

- Access to records may be requested by various bodies, following a major accident, if legal action for negligence is taken.
- Records must be accurate, factual and recorded as soon as possible.

Common accident management

Most First Aid needed in your work will be minor, allowing you time to think carefully before you act. Some procedures for managing major emergencies will also apply to minor injuries.

To reduce cross infection, always wash your own hands thoroughly and use disposable gloves before starting any non-urgent treatment. Try not to cough or breathe over an open wound.

WOUNDS AND BLEEDING

(See also treatment for severe bleeding, page 200.)
When the skin is broken, nature's defensive barrier is damaged and outside infection can enter and blood escape.

Action
- Gently clean the wound, preferably under cool running water. Swab around the wound with sterile gauze. Do not use antiseptics unless this is nursery policy or parents have requested specialist lotions. Leave any obvious clots that may be present.
- Check thoroughly to see there are no fragments, for example glass, grit, or wood splinters in the wound and take out, with tweezers, anything that can be easily removed. If anything is embedded, just leave it and cover the wound gently with a sterile dressing, do not probe and prod.
- If the wound is clean with no debris, place a cotton or linen pad over the cleaned wound and apply pressure.
- Then apply a sterile dressing and bandage it in place. If blood continues to come through, apply a further pad and bandage over the first.
- Raise the area if possible. A sling may be necessary for a cut arm.
- The wound should be re-checked in twelve hours to see if healing has started.
- Further help should be sought if:
  - the wound obviously has debris present
  - the bleeding does not settle
  - the wound looks jagged and the cut edges cannot be brought together
  - signs of infection develop such as the wound not healing, swelling and redness with pain and a discharge of yellow pus.

Grazes

Children frequently fall in playgrounds and scrape their knees. Although minor injuries, they can be particularly painful as the tops of many nerve endings are shorn off. These are often dirty wounds which are difficult to clean.

Action

- Run copious flowing water over the area either by tap or using jugs.
- Pat the graze dry.
- Cover with a non-stick dressing and secure in place with bandage or non-allergenic tape.
- Refer to specialist help if you feel the wound is not clean.
- Watch for signs of infection. If the wound is not healing, there is swelling and redness with pain or a discharge of yellow pus, seek further help.

Nose bleeds

These are common, minor incidents in childhood that are usually harmless and frequently can be left alone. If persistent, the following action can be taken.

Action

- Lean the child forward, give him a bowl or tissue to hold.
- Ask him to pinch the bony area in the middle of his nose.
- Remind him not or blow his nose for several hours after bleeding has stopped.
- Do not plug the nose or put keys down his back to frighten him!

Bruises

Here, the blood vessels have been damaged but the skin is not broken, the bleeding is under the surface causing a bluish discoloration.

Action

- Normally, bruises resolve of their own accord but, if painful, an ice pack can help.
- Raise and support a painful limb.
- Some children with haemophilia, where the blood clotting mechanism is affected, may need medical attention following a bruise.

REMEMBER

- Clots are nature's plasters and are good at sealing small wounds and stopping bleeding, so never remove them.
- Even tiny amounts of blood can go a long way and appear very frightening to a young child, so he will need cuddles and reassurance. Always tell him what is happening.

BONE FRACTURES, BONE INJURIES AND SPRAINS

Children's bones are supple and break only under severe force. However, they can bend or crack.

Fractures may be:

- simple – a break or a crack in a bone
- comminuted – the bone breaks into multiple fragments
- greenstick – (only in children) there is a split in an immature bone.

Fractures may be open or closed.

- In an open fracture, the broken bones are forced through the skin, causing a wound with potential for infection to enter.
- In a closed fracture, the skin remains intact over the break but there may still be damage to surrounding tissue and ligaments.

Signs to indicate a child may have suffered a fracture include:

- obvious deformity
- pain and swelling
- reluctance or difficulty in moving a limb or joint
- the history of the accident, for example a heavy fall from a tree or off a climbing frame onto a hard surface.

Action

- Fully assess the child and follow major accident management (see pages 193–204).
- Do not move the child as you may cause further damage.
- Steady and support the fracture, if necessary with your hands, slings, or rolled blankets.
- Cover open wounds with sterile dressings and control any bleeding.
- Do not give anything to eat or drink.
- All fractures will need hospital treatment.

Suspected fracture of the spine

This is an extremely serious but, luckily, rare injury in young children. The spinal cord, (the major nerve of the body) is protected within the spine by the bony vertebral column. If the back or neck is moved following a break in a vertebra, the cord may be damaged. If this happens permanent loss of sensation and paralysis below the injury site will take place.

Action

- Follow major emergency management (see pages 193–204).
- Keep the child still. Never move a child you suspect to have hurt their neck or back unless there is immediate and obvious danger to his life and you have to perform ABC (see pages 194–199). If this is essential, extra help must be found to support both sides of the head to control and limit neck movement.
- An emergency ambulance should be requested. Full information must be

given to the control unit so that specialist equipment can be sent to immo-bilise the neck or back during his transfer to hospital.

KEY POINT

Shock may occur with any fracture.

Sprains and other related injuries

Sprains are injuries to the ligaments that surround and support joints, and include tearing of the surrounding tissues. Sudden forceful wrenching move-ments are often the cause. Joints usually affected are the ankle joint or, less commonly, the elbow.

Signs are often indistinguishable from fractures and if in doubt always treat as for a break.

Action
- Elevate the limb to avoid extra strain and reduce swelling.
- Support the area. Use a sling for an arm.
- Cold compresses can give pain relief and reduce swelling. Packs of frozen peas can be wrapped around the ankle or elbow joint.

Dislocation

A bone is displaced from its joint with tearing of the surrounding and supporting ligaments by a strong force pulling it into an abnormal position. This is most likely to occur in the shoulder, thumb and finger. The child will have pain, reluc-tance to move the area and the joint will seem abnormal.

Action
- Support the injured area, using a sling for an injured shoulder or hand.
- Transfer the child to hospital.
- Never attempt to try to replace the bone into the socket.

Bony injuries are particularly painful and can distort a child's body image. For example if a child sees his leg at a strange angle, his fear and pain will increase. Explaining what is happening and how it will be made better will help. A young child will need his comfort object.

CHOKING

Small pieces of food and objects such as tiny parts of toys may stick at the back of a child's throat, resulting in blocking or limiting the airway. Obstruction also happens when the throat is irritated and swells. The following reasons explain why choking is more likely in children.
- Children place objects into their mouth for exploration purposes (see chapter 3).

- Swallowing mechanisms in babies are immature, inappropriate food for the developmental stage may be given – especially foods that fragment and are lumpy, and young children often hurry to finish a meal.
- In mixed age group play situations, toddlers may have access to toys dangerous for them such as small construction pieces, beads or buttons.
- Some children with special needs may have prolonged difficulty in swallowing.

Signs to indicate choking are:
- coughing
- gasping for air
- turning red in the face and neck and then blue
- inability to speak or cry
- unconsciousness.

Action – managing a baby who is choking

Remain calm, but act quickly. Remove any obvious obstruction from the baby's mouth with a finger, but do not attempt to clear debris from the back of the throat.

1 Aim to get the baby's head lower than his chest to help gravity.
2 Lay the baby's head downwards on your forearm, supporting his head and chest.
3 Firmly slap the infant between the shoulder blades up to five times.

If this is unsuccessful call for an ambulance.

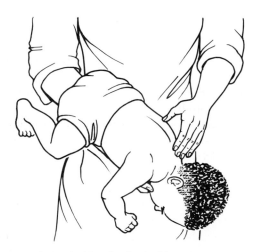

Managing a baby who is choking

4 Turn the baby onto his back.
5 Give up to five chest thrusts using two fingers, pushing downwards onto the breastbone, one every three seconds.
6 Re-check his mouth.

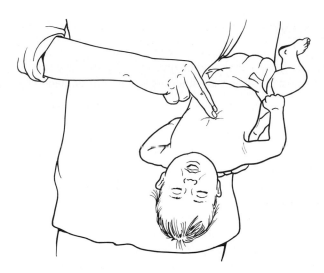

Chest thrusts for a baby

Repeat actions 1 to 6 until an ambulance arrives. Give artificial ventilation if he becomes unconscious (see page 196).

Action – managing a child, one to eight, who is choking

Remain calm, but act quickly. Remove any obvious obstruction from the child's mouth with a finger, but do not attempt to clear debris from the back of the throat. Encourage him to cough.

1 Aim to help gravity by lowering his head below the obstruction, so get him to bend forward.
2 Slap him firmly between the shoulder blades with the heel of your hand up to five times.
3 If back slapping is unsuccessful and the child continues to be unable to breathe, abdominal thrusts may be required.
   - Stand or kneel the child in front of you with his back towards you.
   - Clench your fist and place it against his lower breastbone.
   - Push your clenched fist into his chest with a quick inward upward movement.
   - Repeat up to a total of five times.
   - Check his mouth to see if the obstruction has been dislodged.
   - Give five more back slaps.

If your immediate measures fail to remove the obstruction and his condition deteriorates, you may need to give artificial ventilation and send for immediate medical help.

DO NOT

- poke anything down his throat to try and move the obstruction (use only your finger to clear debris from the front of the mouth)
- use excessive force when slapping either a baby's or toddler's back.

KEY POINTS

- Abdominal thrusts should *never* be performed on babies.
- Preferably, thrusts should be given only by specially trained staff.
- Care must be taken that other organs are not damaged by excessive force.

Inhalation

A flap of skin at the back of the throat, the epiglottis, protects the lungs from inhalation of objects. Occasionally, small, round, smooth articles by-pass the epiglottis and are inhaled directly into the lungs, causing damage. Peanuts, which swell on reaching the lungs, are especially harmful.

Signs may be:

- initial signs of choking which then settle
- wheezy or whistling breath noises
- persistent irritant cough.

Action

- If necessary, treat for choking.
- Seek further medical help to prevent lung damage.

CONVULSIONS

Convulsions take place when a sudden burst of electrical energy occurs in the brain. There are many causes:

- a response to a high temperature, often in children under two and occasionally up to five years
- damage or injury to the brain
- an infection, especially measles or meningitis
- epilepsy.

As well as the causes of convulsions being many so the severity varies. Signs of minor convulsions might include:

- vagueness in the child
- staring of the eyes or blankness
- slight twitching of lips, eyelids or head
- automatic movements.

These minor absences will not usually affect a child's safety and normal good practice of supervision and appropriate activities should keep him safe. However, it is important that further advice is sought to clarify why this is happening

Major convulsions or fits usually occur in three stages.

Stage 1:

- uncontrolled, rapid rise in temperature
- pallor with fixed and staring eyes
- crying out and falling to the ground with a sudden loss of consciousness
- blue lips and dribbling – the child is unable to swallow
- breath holding

- passing urine involuntarily
- muscles becoming rigid, especially the back and neck, and the jaw clamping
- tongue or the inside of the mouth being bitten.

Stage 2:
- body twitching – usually beginning in one place, but often progressing to involve the whole body.

Stage 3:
- the child sleeps or he appears dazed
- he has no memory of the convulsion.

Action
- If you suspect a high temperature, cool the child by tepid sponging, working from the head down. Remember to leave the water to evaporate, do not dry him.
- Clear the area around him so when he twitches or thrashes he will not hurt himself, and keep other children away from the immediate scene.
- Remove his glasses if he wears them.
- When he sleeps, turn him into the recovery position.

Then, proceed with the following.
- Change him if he is wet or soiled.
- Reassure him.
- Supervise him if he appears dazed.
- Inform the parents. This is especially important if this is his first convulsion.
- Record the time and length of the convulsion.
- If he has a history of convulsions, carry out any existing, previously agreed, medical instructions such as giving paediatric Paracetamol to reduce temperature and giving anti-epileptic medication.
- Reassure the other children and explain about convulsions. Tell them they are not serious but can be frightening to watch.

DO NOT

- force anything between the teeth, you could break a tooth and push it down his throat.

If the convulsion is his first, lasts longer than ten minutes, or is one of a series, inform his parents and arrange transfer to hospital.

HEAD INJURY

Any injury to the head is potentially serious, especially if a child has lost consciousness

Breathing and heartbeat can be affected if the head is damaged. Major accidents, falls and shaking of babies, can all cause damage to the delicate brain, encased within the bony skull. A baby has a large head in relation to his body size with immature neck muscles unable to give good head support, so the effects of shaking are increased. If the brain swells and blood vessels are torn, the bones protecting the brain cannot expand and allow the swelling to disperse. Pressure on the brain itself is increased.

Action

- Send for immediate help.
- If the baby is unconscious, follow priorities as for a major accident (see pages 193–204).
- Control any minor bleeding on the scalp, but do not put pressure on any head wounds that show indentation of the skull.

An ambulance should *always* be requested for a child who has hit or banged his head if:

- he has been unconscious for any time at all
- he has a large cut on his head
- there is blood coming out of his ears or nose
- he has a convulsion
- clear fluid leaks from an ear or nose (this may be spinal fluid that surrounds the brain).

Apparently minor head injury

Active groups of children often have head clashes and bumps after falls from such things as climbing frames and bicycles, and usually no harm is done, apart from a bruise or a slight cut. Occasionally, however, a child at first appears unaffected, but slow bleeding under the skull may start and cause a gradual build-up of pressure on the brain. For safety, children should always be monitored for 24 hours following a knock to the head and parents and carers must always be told if a bump to the head happens at school or nursery.

Signs of possible head injury are:

- drowsiness
- sickness and vomiting
- a bad headache several hours after the accident
- a baby may refuse feeds or be fractious
- unequal pupils in the eyes.

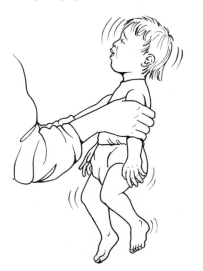

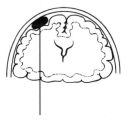

A clot causing pressure
under the skull

Shaking can result in bleeding under the skull, causing pressure on the brain

Action
Seek medical help.

Never shake a baby or young child.

Activity
1 Devise an information sheet for parents and carers whose children attend your nursery. In it, describe the major and minor signs to look for if an accident happens.
2 Devise a check list for monitoring the child during the 24 hours after an injury.

BURNS AND SCALDS

All burns are painful and potentially serious (see pages 201–202).

KEY POINT

Medical help is needed for any burn or scald larger than a 10 pence piece.

POISONING

A poison is a substance which, if taken in sufficient amounts, can cause temporary or permanent damage to a child's health.
Poisons may be:

- swallowed –pills, medicines, berries, alcohol, corrosive substances
- inhaled – solvents, chemical fumes, gas
- absorbed through the skin – garden chemicals
- instilled at the eye – garden sprays
- injected – dangerous drugs.

If poison enter the blood stream it can be carried throughout the body to all tissues, damaging various organs. Signs and symptoms of poisoning will depend on the type of poison, how it entered the body and how long ago it was taken.
Signs of *swallowed* poison may include:

- tummy pains, and vomiting and diarrhoea
- pallor
- drowsiness or unconsciousness
- a slow pulse
- a smell of the substance around the mouth or on the breath, for example alcohol or nail varnish remover
- possible burning around the mouth.

Signs of *inhaled* poison may include:

- irregular and difficult breathing
- gasping for air.

Signs of *absorbed* or *instilled* poisons may include:
- difficulty in breathing
- eye or skin irritation
- rashes
- convulsions.

Signs of *injected* poison may include:
- depression
- abnormal behaviour
- drowsiness or unconsciousness

Action
If the child is unconscious:
- follow priorities in accident emergencies (see pages 193–204)
- check for A B C and place in the recovery position (see pages 194–200)
- seek an emergency ambulance and get samples of possible poison ready for identification.

If the child is conscious:
- get urgent medical help as the full effects of a poison may not be immediately obvious
- if the child is able to talk, ask him what he has taken and how much
- try to keep him calm and still to slow down the spread of the poison
- collect any samples that might be useful in identifying the particular poison such as the remnants of bottles, pills, berries or leaves from any plants. If he has vomited, collect this and take it with you to the hospital
- if there are signs of burning around his mouth, give him sips of plain water or milk to help dilute the poison and gently bathe the area around his mouth
- place him in the recovery position while awaiting the ambulance and check his levels of consciousness. If he stops breathing give artificial respiration.

DO NOT

- attempt to make him sick – if he has swallowed a corrosive substance, this would increase the burning effects when he vomits
- give fluids unless he has burns around his mouth – see above
- distress him by trying to keep him awake, just keep him calm and still.

ALLERGIES

The body's immune system produces antibodies as a reaction to a contact with a usually harmless irritant specific to an individual child. Each contact with the specific irritant increases the body's response. Irritants or 'triggers' can be wide and commonly include pollen, dust mites, chemicals, and certain foods.

Symptoms include:
- itchy eyes and running nose
- coughing
- rashes

- stomach pains
- diarrhoea.

Action

If possible, the trigger should be removed or reduced. Generally, these are minor ailments and resolve as the child reaches puberty. Symptomatic treatment is usually prescribed by the family doctor and this should be given if requested by the parents.

Anaphylaxis

This is an extreme, life threatening, allergic reaction which can occur. Triggers for this are commonly nuts, eggs, fish, especially shell fish, bee and wasp stings and occasionally some antibiotic medicines. Children should wear identification bracelets if they are known to have this reaction.

Signs develop rapidly:
- rash and tingling of the skin
- swelling of the face and throat leading to airway restriction
- increasing difficulty in breathing
- shock and death.

Action

This is a major emergency requiring an immediate response. Seek help from within the setting and call an emergency ambulance.

Children who have had a diagnosed episode of anaphylaxis will have two pre-loaded syringes of adrenalin (EpiPen or Anapen) that should be readily available at all times. School and nursery staff should all know where they are kept. The small, fine needle of the syringe is inserted into a fleshy part of the outer arm or thigh and the drug given. The effect should be immediate. A second dose can be given after five minutes if necessary.

KEY POINTS

In settings where it is known a child is vulnerable to anaphylaxis, a management policy should be developed. All staff need to know how to protect the child and individual staff members should receive training in giving adrenalin which may be life saving.

FOREIGN BODIES

These are small objects that have found their way into the wrong place. It is common in young children, who love to explore and fit fingers and other small things such as beads, toys and pen tops into nooks and crannies in their bodies. Sometimes foreign bodies enter naturally such as insects into ears, or grit and dust into eyes.

In the ears – signs

- The child tells you he has pushed something in.
- A discharge is seen, or a smell comes from his ear.
- His hearing is affected.
- He complains of discomfort or pain.

In the ears – action

- If you can easily see the object at the edge of the ear, gently remove it with tweezers.
- Tilt his head sideways to encourage the object to drop out.
- Seek medical help.

DO NOT

- poke or prod (you may push the object deeper into the ear, or damage the eardrum).

In the nose – signs

- He usually tells you.

In the nose – action

- Tell him to breathe through his mouth.
- Seek medical help.

DO NOT

- tell him to blow his nose (if young, he may inhale pulling the object deeper).

In the eyes – signs

- Where dust, sand and grit are flying around it may be obvious.
- Chemicals may have been splashed over the eye such as bleach.
- Pain and irritation in the eye.
- Watering of the eye.
- An obvious foreign body is embedded.
- His eye has been damaged with a large object (stick or bat for example) during a game.

In the eyes – action

- Stop him from rubbing his eye as this may scratch the delicate cornea.
- Wash the eye out with, preferably, sterile saline solution, otherwise use plenty of tepid water. Using an eye bath or an egg cup, ask him to blink into the cup.
- If this is not possible, tilt his head and run fluid from a jug, starting from the side of the nose. You will need a helper to hold his head still.
- Cover the eye with a sterile pad.
- If the eye continues to be painful, or there is an obvious wound to the eye, seek medical help urgently.
- Reassure him. Injuries to eyes can be both painful and frightening.

KEY POINT

In any accident involving a child, if you are unsure about what to do, always seek a second opinion.

Activity

Research the sources of training in First Aid that are available locally for you.
a) Who organises this training – voluntary bodies, education or health services?
b) How long do these courses last and what is their cost?
c) Where do they take place?
d) Do they offer different levels of training, for example for child care managers or general child care workers?
e) How are they assessed and do they offer a certificate on completion? If the course offers a certificate, for how long is it valid?

First Aid boxes

A First Aid box is a legal requirement for employers under The Health and Safety (First Aid) Regulations 1981. The box itself needs to be waterproof, air tight and readily recognised – normally white with a green cross on the background. Often, nurseries keep a smaller travelling box packed ready to accompany outings.

Both boxes need basic contents and First Aid guidance leaflets. They should be equipped to meet the needs of the children in the setting – amounts and types of dressings and bandages will vary according to the potential need.

First Aid box

Individually wrapped sterile adhesive dressings (assorted sizes)		20
Sterile pads		2
Triangular bandages (preferably sterile)		4
Safety pins		6
Individually wrapped unmedicated wound dressings	12 x 12 cm	6
	18 x 18 cm	2
Disposable gloves (pair)		1
First Aid general guidance leaflet		1

NB The above are the statutory requirements for employers to provide for settings with up to ten employees.

A centre with young children will need additional items including:
Scissors
Tweezers
Non-allergenic tape
Crêpe bandages
Sterile gauze
Form for workers to sign and date when the box was refilled, checked and cleaned.

Travelling First Aid kit	
Individually wrapped, sterile, adhesive dressings	6
Individually wrapped, sterile unmedicated dressings 18 x 18 cm	1
Triangular bandages	2
Safety pins	2
Individually wrapped cleaning wipes	1
Disposable gloves (pair)	1
First Aid general guidance leaflet	1
Plus:	
For early years and pre-school settings, additional items may be required for their specific needs	
Contents checklist with spaces for dating and signing by the person checking the box	

First Aid box contents (required under the Health and Safety (First Aid) Regulations 1981, amended 1997)

A box should be regularly checked for:

- numbers and conditions of dressings
- the dates on dressings to ensure they are still sterile
- cleanliness.

KEY POINT

Medicines, lotions and creams should not be part of a First Aid kit.
Any medicine an individual child needs should be stored in a locked medicine cabinet.

Record keeping

Confidential health records on each child should be kept and stored in a locked cabinet with access limited to essential personnel. However, they must be accessible for emergency use. Standard health records should include the following information.

- Current telephone number for parents and carers, including home and work number with any necessary extension numbers, plus an additional follow-up contact name and number.
- The child's general practitioner's and health visitor's names, addresses and telephone numbers.
- The child's health information sheet with immunisation status, including date of most recent tetanus dose, special health needs including any prescribed medicines, known allergies, and religious and cultural requirements.
- Any written permission given by parents for emergency treatment.

RECORDING ACCIDENTS

See also recording the accident in Severe Emergencies (page 203). All accidents, however minor and including those that happen on outings, must be recorded in an accident book. This record must be made as soon as possible. The information should always include the following details.

- Name of the child.
- Date, time and place of the accident.
- Briefly what happened.
- Description of the injury.
- Name of the person who dealt with the accident.
- The First Aid treatment given.
- Whether additional medical help was sought.
- Some settings use the system of a book and carbon copies so one sheet can be placed in the child's records and a duplicate given to the parents when the child is collected.

Parents must always be notified of any accident. If it is a minor one, then usually the key worker can explain what happened when the child is collected at the end of the session. However, if a child remains distressed, the accident more serious, or medical attention is needed, then parents or carers must be contacted immediately. Parents have a right to be kept fully informed of their child's welfare to allow them to make informed decisions on any actions needed. Remember that, very occasionally, what initially seems a slight injury can lead to unexpected complications.

QUICK CHECKS

1 What is First Aid?
2 When setting up your own day care unit, what decisions would you make about First Aid training for your staff?
3 What ten priorities must you consider when faced with a major accident in the nursery?
4 What are the main differences when giving artificial ventilation to a baby and a child of five?
5 What do you understand by the ABC of First Aid?
6 What are the differences in performing chest compression on a) a baby and b) a child aged up to eight.
7 List the signs of shock and say in what situations it may happen.
8 How would you manage a child who had suffered a severe cut from a kitchen knife and was losing blood rapidly?
9 Describe the main treatment for severe burns.
10 Describe the recovery position and explain why it is important when treating an unconscious child.
11 What information should you have with you if you accompany a child to hospital who has suffered an accident?
12 What might be the differences in managing a) a child with a bleeding wound who has a cut from pushing her hand through a glass window and b) child who has a cut from a knife?

13 What are the signs that a wound is infected?
14 What would you do if a child fell from the climbing frame and was unable to move her neck?
15 List three important safety facts to know before you perform abdominal thrusts on a young child, who is choking.
16 In what situations would you seek immediate hospital transfer for a child having a convulsion?
17 Why is it important to monitor a child for 24 hours following a bang to the head?
18 A four-year-old in your care appears to have swallowed mouthfuls of bleach – what would you do?
19 What standard information should be kept in a child's health records stored at a nursery or school?
20 What are the essential contents of a First Aid box for a pre-school day care setting?

USEFUL ADDRESSES

The Anaphylaxis Campaign
2 Clockhouse Road
Farnborough
Hampshire GU14 7QY
Tel: 01252 54029

British Red Cross Society
9 Grosvenor Crescent
London SW1X 7EJ

Chartered Society of Physiotherapy
14 Bedford Row
London WC1 RED

Child Accident Prevention Trust
4th Floor
Clerks Court
18–20 Farringdon Lane
London EC1R 3AU
Tel: 0207 608 3828

Childline
Tel: (Freefone) 0800 1111

Child Poverty Action Group
4th Floor
1–5 Bath Street
London EC1V 9PY

Council for Disabled Children
8 Wakely Street
London EC1V 7EQ

Disability Resource Team
Pelmark House
11 Amwell End
Ware
Hertfordshire SG12 9HP
Tel: 01920 466005

Foundation for the Study of Infant
Deaths (FSID)
14 Halkin Street
London SW1X 7DP
Tel: 0207 2350965

The Handicapped Adventure
Playground Association (HAPA)
Fulham Palace
Bishop's Avenue
London SW6 6EA
Tel: 01604 79230

Home Start UK
2 Salisbury Road
Leicester LE1 7QR
Tel: 0116 2339955
(Offers support, friendship and practical help at home to families with pre-school children who are experiencing difficulties)

National Association for the
Prevention of Cruelty to Children
(NSPCC)
National Centre
42 Curtain Road
London EC2A 3NH
Tel: (Freefone 24 hour Helpline) 0800 800 500
(Counselling, information and advice to anyone concerned about a child at risk of abuse)

National Association of Toy and
Leisure Libraries
68 Churchway,
London NW1 1LT
Tel: 0207 3874592

National Childminding Association
8 Masons Hill
Bromley
Kent BR2 9EY
Tel: 0208 4646164

National Playbus Association
Unit G
Amos Castel Estate
Junction Road
Brislington
Bristol BS4 5AG

Parentline UK
Endway House
The Endway
Hadleigh
Benfleet
Essex SS7 2AN
Tel: (Helpline) 01702 559900
(Helpline for parents and carers under
stress)

Royal Society for the Prevention of
Accidents
The Safety Centre
353 Bristol Road
Birmingham B5 7ST
Tel: 0121 2482000

Serene (including CRY-SIS Helpline)
London WC1N 3XX
Tel: (CRY-SIS Helpline) 0207 4045011
(Support for parents and carers deal-
ing with excessive crying, demanding
behaviour and sleep problems)

The Terence Higgins Trust
52–54 Gray's Inn Road
London WC1X 8JU
Tel: 0207 6274594

INDEX

Page references in *italics* indicate illustrations, figures or tables.